"*Sinus Relief Now* is a unique contribution t[...] with treating the patient as a whole. Dr. Jo[...] flammatory process applies to the diseases of [...] ing, sleep apnea, and acid reflux, and what you can do for it. He has gone past simply recommending more antibiotics. I believe anyone with these conditions will profit by reading this fine book."

—Murray Grossan, M.D., author of *The Sinus Cure*
and inventor of the Hydro Pulse Nasal/Sinus Irrigation System

"If you suffer with sinus problems, allergies, or asthma you must read this book. This informative and authoritative guide provides the insights that can change your health. By exploring alternative and traditional treatments, Dr. Josephson provides a comprehensive approach which brings together the best of both worlds. He clearly explains the synergy between Eastern and Western medicine, providing lasting treatment options for sinus disease, allergies, asthma, snoring, sleep apnea, and reflux esophagitis (GERD)."

—Richard Firshein, D.O., author of *Reversing Asthma*
and *Your Asthma-Free Child*

"As a leading publisher of all kinds of health information, I have seen it all. And Dr. Josephson's new way of connecting the seemingly unrelated health concerns that millions of people experience every day, *Sinus Relief Now*, is the single most valuable sourcebook for patients and physicians on treating the patient as a whole. Dr. Josephson's coining of the term *CAID* (chronic airway-digestive inflammatory disease) is ingenious because CAID affects millions of people, many of whom are still searching for the answers to their problems. *Sinus Relief Now* will help these patients greatly. It is about time that a physician has written about the inflammatory process that causes sinus, allergy, asthma, bronchitis, snoring, sleep apnea, and GERD, and treats them holistically."

—Martin Edelston, Founder and President, Boardroom Inc.,
publishers of *Bottom Line/Personal* and *Bottom Line/Health*

continued . . .

Sinus Relief Now

THE GROUNDBREAKING
5-STEP PROGRAM FOR SINUS, ALLERGY,
AND ASTHMA SUFFERERS

Jordan S. Josephson, M.D.

A PERIGEE BOOK

A PERIGEE BOOK
Published by the Penguin Group
Penguin Group (USA) Inc.
375 Hudson Street, New York, New York 10014, USA
Penguin Group (Canada), 90 Eglinton Avenue East, Suite 700, Toronto, Ontario M4P 2Y3, Canada
(a division of Pearson Penguin Canada Inc.)
Penguin Books Ltd., 80 Strand, London WC2R 0RL, England
Penguin Group Ireland, 25 St. Stephen's Green, Dublin 2, Ireland (a division of Penguin Books Ltd.)
Penguin Group (Australia), 250 Camberwell Road, Camberwell, Victoria 3124, Australia
(a division of Pearson Australia Group Pty. Ltd.)
Penguin Books India Pvt. Ltd., 11 Community Centre, Panchsheel Park, New Delhi—110 017, India
Penguin Group (NZ), Cnr. Airborne and Rosedale Roads, Albany, Auckland 1310, New Zealand
(a division of Pearson New Zealand Ltd.)
Penguin Books (South Africa) (Pty.) Ltd., 24 Sturdee Avenue, Rosebank, Johannesburg 2196, South Africa

Penguin Books Ltd., Registered Offices: 80 Strand, London WC2R 0RL, England

While the author has made every effort to provide accurate telephone numbers and Internet addresses at the time of publication, neither the publisher nor the author assumes any responsibility for errors, or for changes that occur after publication. Further, the publisher does not have any control over and does not assume any responsibility for author or third-party websites or their content.

First edition: December 2006

Library of Congress Cataloging-in-Publication Data

Josephson, Jordan S.
    Sinus relief now : the groundbreaking 5-step program for sinus, allergy, and asthma sufferers / Jordan S. Josephson.
        p. cm.
    "A Perigee Book."
    Includes index.
    ISBN 0-399-53298-6
    1. Sinusitis—Treatment—Popular works. 2. Allergy—Treatment—Popular works. 3. Asthma—Treatment—Popular works. I. Title.
    RF354.J67 2006
    616.2'1206—dc22

                                                                                    2006026280

PRINTED IN THE UNITED STATES OF AMERICA

10 9 8 7 6 5 4 3 2 1

PUBLISHER'S NOTE: Neither the publisher nor the author is engaged in rendering professional advice or services to the individual reader. The ideas, procedures, and suggestions contained in this book are not intended as a substitute for consulting with your physician. All matters regarding your health require medical supervision. Neither the author nor the publisher shall be liable or responsible for any loss or damage allegedly arising from any information or suggestion in this book.

The recipes contained in this book are to be followed exactly as written. The publisher is not responsible for your specific health or allergy needs that may require medical supervision. The publisher is not responsible for any adverse reactions to the recipes contained in this book.

Most Perigee Books are available at special quantity discounts for bulk purchases for sales promotions, premiums, fundraising, or educational use. Special books, or book excerpts, can also be created to fit specific needs. For details, write: Special Markets, The Berkley Publishing Group, 375 Hudson Street, New York, New York 10014.

In loving memory of my grandparents, Julius and Faye Goldstein and Joseph and Esther Josephson, and my father-in-law, Arthur Wantuch.

ACKNOWLEDGMENTS

There are many important people I would like to thank that have each helped, in his or her own way, in the creation of this book. I am grateful for the scientific knowledge shared with me by many of my medical colleagues, including Yosef Krespi, M.D.; Tibian Abramovitz, M.D.; David Sherris, M.D.; Eugene Kern, M.D.; Carolyn Sierra, M.D.; Elena Ferran, M.D.; Robert Altman, M.D.; Winston Vaughn, M.D.; Paul Miller, D.D.S.; Donald Chalfin, M.D.; Murray Grossan, M.D.; and Gary Josephson, M.D. Last, I would like to extend a special thanks to Seth Rosenberg, M.D., without whom this book could not have been written.

On the Eastern medical front, I am indebted to Alex Kulick, M.D., and Amy Josephson, D.C. I continue to learn everyday from my pharmaceutical allies, including Paul Feingertz, R.Ph.; Lisa Charneski, Pharm.D., B.C.P.S.; and the great folks at Goldberger's Pharmacy in New York City.

Throughout my career, I have been fortunate to work with many great physicians. I am indebted to my mentors Charles R. Greene, M.D.; Michael J. Zinner, M.D.; Allan L. Abramson, M.D.; Michael E. Johns, M.D.; and David W. Kennedy, M.D. and all the others who have taught me. I am also grateful for the opportunity that I have had to teach all over the world, and share my thoughts regarding CAID and sinus disease.

The emotional support I have received from my family and friends has been overwhelming. My wife, Mara; daughter, Jaclyn; and sons, Julius and Jared, all know that they are my light. I am a very lucky man to have them in my life. I am ever thankful for the love and devotion I have always received from my parents, Sheila and Stanley Josephson. I thank my siblings Mark, Amy, and Gary for their love and constant support throughout my life.

I offer special thanks to my professional team that has worked so hard in putting this book together. My office staff has been wonderful during the entire writing process. I am grateful for the help that Janice Cedeno and Eslyn Roman continue to provide for both me and my patients. I would like to thank Kim Urdahl for helping me with making my edits. Pam Liflander's literary skills and insights helped me bring my thoughts and ideas to these pages. Carol Mann, my agent, was able to find me the best publisher for this project. Christel Winkler, Jeanette Shaw, and John Duff at Perigee have been extraordinary. Ian Rogers has provided the most fantastic artwork for this book.

Finally, I want to thank my patients. For more than 20 years, they have helped me understand these disease processes better through their own experiences. I thank them for allowing me to treat them and for letting me share their problems with a broader audience so that others may learn from both their ordeals and their triumphs.

CONTENTS

PART THREE: COMPLETING SINUS RELIEF

INTRODUCTION

More than 70 million Americans suffer from sinus disease, allergies, and asthma, and 25 percent of the population snore or suffer from sleep apnea. If you are one of these people, you may share many of their symptoms, ranging from mildly annoying to severely painful and debilitating: postnasal drip, nasal stuffiness and obstruction, headaches, coughing, sore throat, swollen glands, hoarseness, mouth breathing, decreased sense of smell and/or taste, facial or dental pain, ear pressure, dark circles under the eyes, wheezing, dizziness, high- or low-grade fevers, sweats or hearing loss. You might not be sleeping well, which can lead to recurring fatigue. Your snoring may keep your spouse or partner awake at night, leaving him or her tired as well.

You may have decided to neglect your symptoms, chalking them up as some of the more mundane nuisances to an otherwise healthy life. You may mistake them as normal signs of aging or are resigned to the fact that these symptoms are somewhat acceptable. Worse, you may not even realize that your senses of smell or taste have diminished. Yet all of these points of view could not be farther from the truth. These are all interconnected symptoms of an increasingly growing health problem and, if left untreated, can result in serious illness. Furthermore, because your problem is complex, it requires careful attention, proper diagnosis and a targeted treatment plan.

If you have tried to address your symptoms, your physician may have been able to provide temporary or minimal relief. Others like you have seen numerous physicians and practitioners to no avail, only to receive inadequate treatment, or worse, have been told just to "live with these symptoms."

I do not believe that any of these scenarios are acceptable. We are all entitled to achieve total health, and if you feel miserable suffering from these symptoms, you deserve to find a solution. I have written this book to teach you how to work with your physician(s) so that together you can come up with a treatment plan that is right for you: one that will give you maximal relief while controlling your problems.

Sinus Disease Affects the Entire Body

The latest research has shown that sinus disease, allergies, and asthma are intimately connected. In addition, sufferers often complain of gastro-esophageal reflux disease (GERD), laryngopharyngeal reflux disease (LPRD), and/or snoring or have sleep apnea. I have recently coined the term *chronic airway-digestive inflammatory disease* (CAID) to describe this very complex set of problems that are often misdiagnosed. CAID directly affects the upper respiratory system (the nose and the sinuses) as well as the lower airway (the lungs) and the gastrointestinal (GI) tract. An inflammatory response in the airway can be initiated by bacteria, viruses, fungi (molds), pollutants, or other irritants, or an allergen. These inflammatory responses can cause a multitude of reactions: The membranes that line the nose, sinuses, and lungs are so sensitive that inflammation in any of these areas can ultimately affect the others. For example, allergies often exacerbate sinus problems, and asthma can be triggered, or is often worsened, by chronic sinus infections. Reflux is often closely associated as both a cause and an effect of this disease process.

CAID also affects many other organs beyond the respiratory (breathing) and digestive systems. For instance, CAID can be linked to heart disease, stroke, infertility, painful headaches, and chronic fatigue syndrome. Each of these conditions can be resolved—or at least properly treated—once CAID has been correctly diagnosed. Along with CAID, I have developed a new paradigm for medicine to diagnose and treat this complex illness. I call it "the Sinus Revolution." It highlights the need for a partnership between you and all of the physicians who may be treating each of the different aspects of this disease process independently. Together, you can address the complex set of symptoms and form a more accurate diagnosis. Ultimately, this will lead to formulating a treatment plan to help you finally begin to feel better.

The Functional Endoscopic Sinus Approach

Sinus and nasal surgery has gone through its own revolution in many ways. I follow and support a technical approach to treating CAID, whose core feature includes functional endoscopic sinus surgery (FESS). This is not just a surgical technique but a medical philosophy based on the tools used to diagnose and treat a host of sinus-related symptoms. It also allows for Eastern and Western remedies to integrate, providing comprehensive treatment from a multitude of resources. This combined approach has distinct advantages. First, practitioners are able to make a more accurate diagnosis and thus are able to treat the five limbs of CAID: sinus disease, allergies, asthma, GERD/LPRD, and snoring/sleep apnea with a more sophisticated medical plan before surgery is even considered. Second, it allows for individuals to take an active role in their treatment, becoming an integral part of the team. Without your help, we as practitioners can do very little.

The medical techniques used in FESS have become a big part of the Sinus Revolution. The success of FESS has brought about a recent increase in interest in the study of sinus disease. Furthermore, this study has brought about a more coordinated approach among the different specialists treating sinus disease, allergies, asthma, GERD/LPRD, snoring, and sleep apnea.

How This Book Works

If you suffer from any of the conditions or symptoms I've just described, there are new grounds for hope. For the first time, you will be able to take control of your sinus disease, allergies, asthma, GERD/LPRD, and/ or snoring/sleep apnea and find the combination of treatments that can restore your health.

As an ear, nose, and throat specialist (a board-certified otolaryngologist), I see—and treat—these issues every day. Personally, I am also a sufferer and have been affected by these symptoms my entire life. However, by following my protocol, I am feeling better than ever. This book is based on my experience with my patients and my own health and is written for the millions of sufferers, who like you, are looking for lasting relief.

The first part of the book deals with your anatomy and explains how your airway functions under the best of circumstances. Next, I explore the different signs and symptoms that you may be experiencing and show how many of them are intimately linked. Then, you'll find a detailed quiz so that you can determine exactly what is troubling you and to what extent your problem is affecting your overall quality of life. With this knowledge, you will be able to pinpoint exactly which aspect of CAID is making you feel sick, so that you will know with confidence what you need to do about it. It will confirm for you whether you are suffering from sinus disease, allergies, asthma, GERD/LPRD, or snoring/sleep apnea or a combination of these.

The second section of the book describes each of the limbs of CAID in detail and discusses the latest treatments for each. I present a full range of options, which include over-the-counter remedies, holistic medicines and allopathic treatments, prescription medications, surgery, and lifestyle changes. I have learned that the best results come from a combination of therapies. In my practice, I often add alternative Eastern practices to the traditional Western medicines and surgery that I perform. These Eastern practices include homeopathy, chiropractic, acupuncture, osteopathy, and mesotherapy, each provided by a specialist who works as part of the treatment team. Many of these practitioners rely on a comprehensive elimination diet so that patients can determine if certain foods are adversely affecting their health. Scientists are now discovering that mold is a major cause of these symptoms, creating an inflammatory response that not only upsets the respiratory system but also affects the digestive tract and the entire body. This issue affects your health and your home or workplace.

Just as one treatment will not fit all people, there are certain groups of people whose special needs require unique treatment. There is a chapter devoted to special-needs individuals who are often affected by sinus problems. Such people include frequent travelers; scuba divers; and those who are also dealing with other chronic illnesses such as AIDS, autoimmune diseases, diabetes, and cancer. I also address the special requirements of children, pregnant women, and the elderly.

When all other options have been tried, it may be necessary to perform surgery. In my practice, I use the latest tools and techniques. I was lucky enough to begin my surgical training during a time when sinus surgery was dramatically changing. The new FESS techniques are less invasive and offer better results than older techniques, and FESS can often be performed right in a doctor's office. When hospitalization is necessary, surgery is usually performed under local anesthesia with sedation, bleeding is minimal, and there is rarely any swelling or black-and-blue marks. Packing is rarely required, and pain is minimal. My patients are usually released from the hospital the same day; most remark that they are immediately breathing easier. Most are back to work the next working day. If you have previously had medical treatment or sinus surgery that did not yield great results, it may be time to consider the next wave of medical care, which should put you back on the road to better overall health.

A Five-Step Plan

Unfortunately, CAID is a chronic disease that will never be cured. However, you can learn to control your symptoms, alleviating unnecessary pain, and responding rapidly to the next episode. This knowledge and an action plan are just as important as recognizing and treating your initial symptoms.

The core of the Sinus Revolution is a simple five-step action plan that anyone can follow. The five steps include making some lifestyle changes and adding new routines to your daily rituals. By abiding by these guidelines, you not only will feel better during the course of your treatment but will find that your symptoms will be easy to control for years to come. I am sure you will agree that such results are worth the effort.

Complete directions for each step of the five-step plan are located throughout this book. They are:

- Learning to take care of your sinuses through proper irrigation
- Managing your environment, including guidelines for limiting mold, allergens, and other pollutants in the home, office, and car
- Nutritional information to help you identify foods that all CAID sufferers need to avoid and to identify foods that trigger *your* CAID symptoms
- A medication (both traditional and holistic) plan that must be followed religiously before, during, and after longer courses of treatment and/or surgery
- Tips for enjoying the progress made and embracing the changes that come with experiencing total health

The Sinus Revolution Promise

I have written this book for the millions of sufferers, and their physicians, because I believe that we are all entitled to live our lives to the fullest. I understand firsthand how CAID affects us every day, and I know how miserable it feels to deal with this disease process. I also know how much better I feel, and how much better my patients feel, once we understand how pervasive our problem is and how to treat it.

With this knowledge, you will be able to speak with your physician in an informed, intelligent manner and become part of the team to find the right treatments for your unique problems. The key to better health lies within this conversation. Doctors are only as good as the information they receive. Therefore, share your newfound knowledge about your illness, the latest treatment options, and their results, with your physician so he or she can be better able to relieve your symptoms, letting you finally enjoy all that the world has to offer.

Here's to you and to better health in your future.

PART ONE

HOW YOUR SINUSES WORK

CHAPTER 1

ANATOMY OF A HEALTHY BODY

At first glance, the nose seems like such a small, insignificant part of the body. It doesn't pump blood, like the heart. It doesn't think and reason, like the brain. It doesn't aid in reproduction, nor does it digest food.

Yet the nose is its own perfect structure, and its components are just as important as those other vital organs for keeping each of us alive. Without the nose, we would not be able to take in oxygen effectively, and the rest of our life-support systems, including the heart and the brain could not function. Our sense of smell and taste, both controlled by the nose, directs us to the nourishment that keeps our stomach functioning properly. These senses also warn us of impending danger, if we start to eat rancid food, or worse, if we come into contact with a life-threatening stench, such as toxic chemicals, smoke, or fire.

From an aesthetic point of view, the nose forms the center of our face and contributes to our unique appearance. In fact, our face and nose can influence another person's opinion of us, even before we speak. When we speak, the nose and the sinuses add a tonal quality to our words. And when we smile, our nose accents this gesture with nasal motion. All of these subtleties support the overall impression we give to people on a daily basis, and contribute to developing our personality and self-esteem.

The nose plays an integral part in many of our biological functions. Of all of its roles, the most important facet of the nose is the ability to take in air. In order for us to survive, the air we breathe needs to be transported to the lungs and then to the brain via the bloodstream. But not just any air will do. For every person, whether they live in coldest Alaska, the tropics of Florida, the Nevada desert or the Louisiana humidity, the air from the outside world needs to be cleaned, heated, and humidified to the exact same temperature and humidity before the body can use it. The air that reaches our lungs has to be regulated to near normal body temperature: between 96.8° and 98.6°F. The ideal humidity is between 75 and 80 percent.

If the nose is not performing these tasks, the rest of the body will not function optimally.

How Air Travels through the Nose

The nose is made up of several bones and soft tissue. When we breathe in through our nose, our lungs are automatically engaged in what is called nasal resistance, the force that the lungs pull on to draw air into our bodies. For the lungs to work optimally, the nose and sinuses have to provide perfect resistance, which is enabled through their unique design.

The tip of the nose is flexible and made of two cartilages (called the upper and lower lateral cartilages), and the upper part of the nose is made of bone (Diagram 1). The middle part of the nose consists of a wall that separates the nose into two discrete sides. This wall, or partition, is called the nasal septum. The front portion of the septum is cartilage, and this part of the nose is flexible. The back third of the septum is bone. The nasal septum is not the only wall that is housed in the nose. There are many septae (plural for septum), or walls, that divide the sinuses.

On each side of the nasal septum exists a nasal passageway, made up of five areas, the most critical being the nasal valve (Diagram 2). The

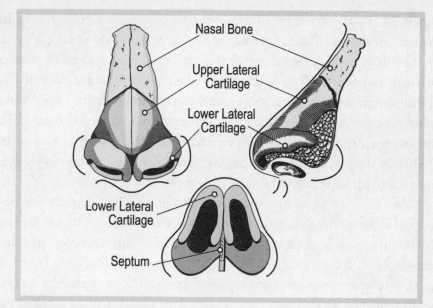

Diagram 1 Anatomy of the nose.

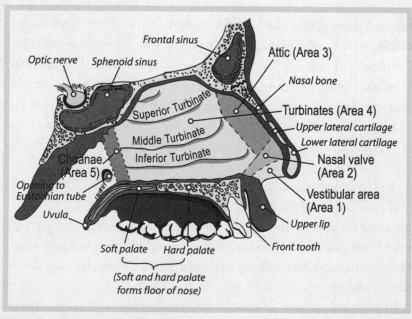

Diagram 2 The nasal passageway.

nasal valve is a triangle formed where the cartilaginous septum meets the junction of the two lateral cartilages, the upper and lower lateral cartilages. This triangle of cartilage forms the narrowest and most critical area for the passage of air within your nose and is flexible. When you pinch the tip of your nose, you close the nasal valve. As the nasal valve closes, you can appreciate the nasal blockage that occurs, cutting off a significant amount of your nasal airway. When this area is closed naturally or as a result of trauma, scarring, or infection, it becomes significantly difficult to breathe through your nose.

When any or all of the five areas of the nasal passageway are obstructed, the air flow through the nose becomes blocked. The magnitude of nasal obstruction depends on which area or combination of areas are affected and the extent to which each of these areas is blocked. The first, the vestibular area is located at the tip of the nose, at the entrance behind the nostrils. The second area is the nasal valve. The third area is called the attic, which lies between the septum and the nasal bones. Area four is located between the septum and the turbinates. Area five, called the choana, lies between the septum and the back of the nose.

A straight nasal septum allows for good air flow. When it is deviated or crooked, the septum can significantly obstruct breathing, limiting our air intake. The extent of the decrease in airflow depends on the amount and location of the deviation. For instance, a major deviation in the back of the nose may not cause as much obstruction as a deviation in the nasal valve area. Typically, blockage in any of these areas will reduce the airflow through the nose, and it will become necessary for you to breathe partially through your mouth to get enough air into your lungs.

THE TURBINATES

As air passes through the nose, it gets heated by finger-like projections called turbinates. Turbinates are bony structures that act as baffles, directing the passage of air along a specific path. The turbinates also act as radiators, adding warm, moist heat to the air as it passes. They also help increase the surface area of the nose to make the heating and humidification process more efficient (Diagrams 3a and 3b).

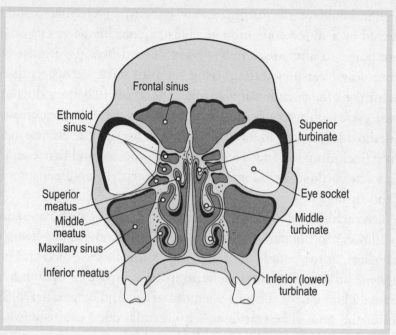

Diagram 3a A frontal view of the face, showing the turbinates.

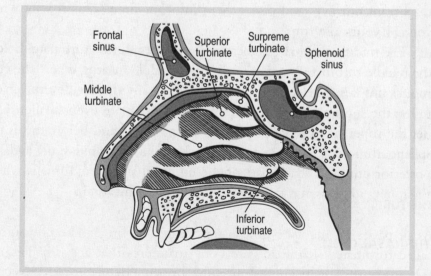

Diagram 3b A side view of the face, showing the turbinates.

The bones of the turbinates are encased in vascular tissue that is covered by a mucous membrane. This vascular tissue swells or shrinks in response to alterations in the body's blood flow. Positional changes (lying down versus standing, lying on your back versus lying on one side or the other), endocrine changes (hormonal changes during menstrual cycles, puberty, menopause, pregnancy, or aging), increased carbon dioxide intake, alterations in blood flow, or even normal daily living (including the foods and fluids that you eat and drink and medicines that you may be taking for other ailments) can affect the swelling of this tissue.

On each side of the nose there are three sets of turbinates: the inferior (lower) turbinates, the middle turbinates, and the superior (upper) turbinates. Some people are born with a fourth set called the supreme (highest) turbinates. Below each turbinate is a space or opening, called a meatus. The inferior turbinates are the largest and lie parallel to the bottom of the nose. The tear duct (nasolacrimal duct) drains into the area below the inferior turbinate, called the inferior meatus. The nasolacrimal duct connects the inside of the eye with the nose. It carries tears from our eyes and passes them into our nose. This is why when you cry your nose runs.

The middle turbinate is located above the inferior turbinate. Below the middle turbinate is a space called the middle meatus, where the ethmoid sinus lies. The superior turbinate is usually the smallest turbinate, unless the supreme turbinates are present, which are even smaller. Under the superior turbinate is the superior meatus and below this is the sphenoethmoidal recess (a space between the sphenoid sinus and the posterior ethmoid (back part of the ethmoid sinus), and this is where the sphenoid sinus and the posterior ethmoid sinus drain.

THE NASAL CYCLE

The turbinates help control air flow by a predetermined pattern of swelling and constricting. The turbinates swell one side of the nose while the other side shrinks. This pattern is called the nasal cycle, and it repeats itself every 2 or 3 hours, all day long. When the nasal cycle is working properly, we are breathing through only one side of the nose at a time, while the other side rests.

At night, the nasal cycle influences the side of the body you choose to sleep on. You may have thought, or even felt, that fluid flows from one side of your face to the other. In actuality, fluid from one side of your nose cannot move to the other side through the septum. Instead, you're experiencing the nasal cycle at work. Some scientists believe that the nasal cycle is what causes most people to turn from side to side when they sleep. Others argue that turning is what causes the nasal cycle to occur. However, we do know that the nasal cycle occurs even when you are wide-awake and standing. So day or night, we breathe through one side of our nose at a time, and it alternates from side to side. The nasal cycle is natural, so most people do not realize their breathing is asymmetric unless there is underlying nasal obstruction.

THE PARANASAL SINUSES

After passing over the turbinates, air travels through the sinuses, which are open pockets or cavities that surround the nose. The sinuses are covered by membranes that respond to the constantly changing environment.

The sinuses clean and prepare the air so that it reaches the lungs free of contaminated particles. They remove pollution (e.g., dirt, dust, or car exhaust), inflammatory agents (e.g., toxins, chemicals, or smoke), allergens (e.g., pollen, ragweed, or mold) and infections (e.g., bacteria, fungi, or viruses) that may be carried in the air.

Most people develop four pairs of sinuses: the ethmoid sinuses, which lie behind the bridge of the nose and between the eye sockets; the frontal sinuses, in the forehead; the maxillary sinuses, located in the cheeks below each eye and above the upper teeth; and the sphenoid sinuses, which are behind the nose and eyes and underneath the brain (Diagram 4). Usually, we are born with only ethmoid and maxillary sinuses. The remaining two pairs develop out of the ethmoid sinuses as

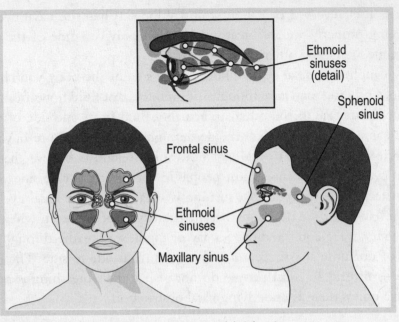

Diagram 4 The four pairs of paranasal sinuses and their locations.

we grow older. By the time we are teenagers and the rest of our bodies have physically matured, the sinuses should be fully developed.

The sizes of each of these pairs of sinuses vary, and some people have significant asymmetries within any of these pairs. One could have large or small sinuses, and some people are even missing a particular pair of sinuses or a single sinus. In fact, the sinus anatomy is so variable it is almost like a fingerprint: You can actually tell people apart based on their particular sinus pattern. As many as 15 percent of all people fail to develop one or more of their sinuses. However, people can exist quite nicely without all of them, and may live their lives without knowing that they do not have a full complement of sinuses.

THE ETHMOID SINUSES

The ethmoid sinuses are the key to nasal health. Just as all roads lead to Rome, mucus produced in any of the sinuses is eventually drained through or by the ethmoid sinuses. For example, the mucus produced in the frontal sinuses drains through the ethmoid sinus by a connection called the frontal duct or frontal recess. The maxillary sinuses drain through an opening called the maxillary ostium. This drains into a funnel-like area called the infundibulum, which is also connected to the ethmoid sinus. From any source, the mucus then passes through the ethmoid sinuses and into the back of the nose.

The front of the ethmoid sinuses sits below the middle turbinate in the middle meatus. The back of the ethmoids sit below the superior turbinate in the superior meatus. The middle turbinate attaches to the outside wall of the sinus, which also serves as the inside wall of the eye. The wall that is created by this attachment is called the ground lamella and separates the anterior and the posterior ethmoid sinus cells.

The ethmoid sinuses are shaped like a beehive and are composed of approximately 22 smaller cavities or cells. Each cavity increases the surface area so that the air can be quickly heated, vaporized, humidified, and filtered as it passes over the mucous blanket that coats the ethmoid sinuses.

THE FRONTAL SINUSES

The frontal sinuses are located in the forehead over the eyes, right behind the eyebrows. They develop after birth around the age of 2, and they achieve full size by the time we are 12. Fully developed frontal sinuses came in a variety of sizes and are not symmetrical from one side of the face to the other. These sinuses are empty air sacks that not only aid in the filtering process but also act as shock absorbers, protecting your brain from any frontal trauma.

THE MAXILLARY SINUSES

The maxillary, or cheek, sinuses are fairly well developed at birth, although they will become larger as the rest of the body continues to grow. The maxillary sinuses are housed in the cheekbones. The roof of the maxillary sinus forms the floor of the space, called the orbit, that houses the eyeball. The floor of the maxillary sinus forms part of the hard palate. Both baby and adult teeth in your upper jaw form in this area. As the teeth drop down, they push through the floor of the maxillary sinus into the mouth. The nerve that feeds into your teeth, your cheeks, and the maxillary sinus is the trigeminal or cranial nerve V. This nerve runs through the roof of the maxillary sinus and provides sensation to your facial skin.

THE SPHENOID SINUSES

The sphenoid sinuses are normally located behind the ethmoid, although in some cases the posterior ethmoid can wrap around the sphenoid. The sphenoid sinuses lie just below the brain and almost in the center of the head. The two sphenoid sinuses are separated by another bony wall or partition, called a septum (Diagram 5). The sphenoid sinuses are barely visible at birth and begin to develop between the ages of 2 and 3 years. They continue to grow throughout childhood, and fully mature by the age of 18. At their largest, they are about the size of a marble.

The sphenoid sinuses have many important structures around them.

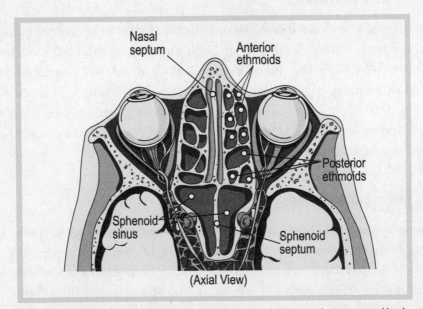

Diagram 5 The sphenoid sinuses are located just below the brain and are separated by the sphenoid septum.

The carotid artery, which carries the blood supply to the brain, travels along each outside wall of the sphenoid sinus. In about 15 percent of the population, this wall is absent and the artery actually sits in the sphenoid sinus. This is known as a dehiscent carotid artery. The optic nerve, which carries visual signals from the eye to the brain, travels through the roof of the sphenoid sinus. Behind the sphenoid sinuses is the cavernous sinus, the vein that drains the blood away from the brain. The pituitary gland, which is responsible for many of your hormone levels, sits above the back part of the roof of the sphenoid sinuses.

More Than You Ever Wanted to Know about Mucus

The major function of the sinuses is to heat, humidify, and clean the air we breathe so that it arrives at the lungs ready for the rest of the body to use. The sinuses complete all of these tasks through the creation of mucus, the sticky substance we usually pay attention to only when we are sick and our bodies seem to be producing too much. In reality, the sinuses constantly produce a significant amount of mucus, whether we are sick or not.

The sinuses normally produce between 1 and 2 liters of mucus per day. Mucus is made up of 95 percent water and has a slightly acidic pH. Healthy mucus is usually clear and watery, but it can become thickened and viscous when we are experiencing an infection. When we are sick or are suffering from allergies, mucus production increases. When your body produces this thicker mucus, you may experience the feeling of postnasal drip. This term is misleading, because normal, healthy mucus is always dripping down into your throat, but you are not aware of it. It is only when the mucus becomes thickened because of an infection that you notice its existence.

Mucus adds moisture to the air taken in through the nose so the lungs receive air with the proper humidity. It also lubricates the membranes of our nose. Mucus contains salts and glycoproteins, which create a barrier to infection. Each set of sinuses are lined by mucous membranes that are covered by a mucous blanket. As air passes through the sinuses, the mucous blanket traps tiny particles, including dirt, chemicals, irritants, dust, pollution, allergens, fungi, molds, viruses, and bacteria. This mechanism allows the dirt to be separated from the air that enters the lungs. These particles attach to the mucus, which is later expelled from the body. It is estimated that the mucous blanket is totally replaced in the nose every 10 to 20 minutes and in the sinuses every 10 to15 minutes.

MUCUS AND THE IMMUNE SYSTEM

When an infectous agent enters our breathing system, the body automatically raises its temperature, and the consistency of the mucus changes: The pH changes, becoming more acidic, and the viscosity or thickness increases. This affects many bodily functions, possibly including a woman's menstrual cycle and her ability to conceive.

Mucus contains immunoglobulins, which are proteins that act as antibodies to defend against bacteria, viruses, and molds. It is secreted along with other infection-fighting substances that make up our immune system. The main goal of the immune system is to identify harmful, foreign substances that enter the body. These can be microorganisms that cause infections (bacteria, fungi, or viruses), antigens (particles that create an allergic response), or particles that can cause inflammation (e.g., pollution). When the body comes into contact with any of these foreign substances, it will elicit a reaction to rid the body of it.

The immune system is a made up of many intricate and multifunctioning systems that work together to fight infection throughout the body, including in your sinuses and nasal cavities. It can be broken down into four basic components:

- Humoral immunity, which produces antibodies from white blood cells (B cells in particular) that fight against bacteria and the antigens that play a role in allergic reactions
- Cell-mediated immunity, which uses white blood cells (T cells) that protect us against viruses and fungi as well as assisting the humoral arm to fight bacteria

- Phagocytic immunity, which causes a cascade of reactions that help the body fight bacteria
- The complement arm, which is made up of bacteria-killing proteins

The humoral arm of the immune system creates antibodies, which bind to antigens and lead to the eventual removal of the offending toxin, bacteria, parasite, or other foreign substance. These antibodies are divided into five main classes of immunoglobulins: immunoglobulin G (IgG), immunoglobulin M (IgM), immunoglobulin A (IgA), immunoglobulin E (IgE), and immunoglobulin D (IgD). Our body fights off infection by producing these immunoglobulins in the right quantity and at the right time to help us survive the constant exposure to environmental antigens. A deficiency in the production of immunoglobulins can lead to serious infections.

IgG is by far the most abundant and plays an important role in preventing allergens from initiating an allergic reaction. IgM is involved in the initial response to an infection as well as with some autoimmune diseases, such as rheumatoid arthritis. IgM also helps the complement arm of the immune system fight infection. IgA is found in tears, saliva, and nasal secretions. This immunoglobulin exhibits a potent antiviral activity that prevents viruses from binding to our respiratory pathway. IgE is present in small quantities but plays a large role in allergic responses. Although all of us produce IgE, those who have allergies seem to overproduce this agent.

WHERE MUCUS COMES FROM

The cavities of the sinuses are lined with mucous membranes, or tissues, that look like the inside of your mouth. These membranes are smooth and shiny and made up of various distinct types of cells. First, a layer of goblet cells produce the mucus through tiny tubes, forming the mucous blanket. These goblet cells are interspersed between hair-like cells called ciliated columnar cells, which move the mucus across the surface of the membrane (Diagram 6). The membranes of all the sinuses are covered

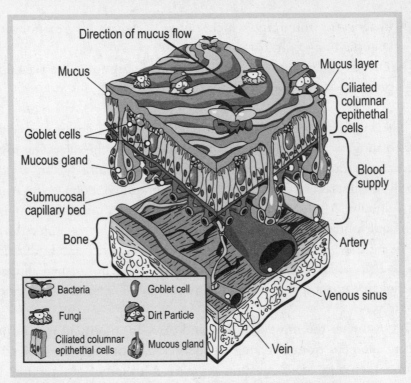

Diagram 6 The layers of the mucous membrane, and the irritants that it traps.

with these ciliated columnar cells. Together, the mucous membranes, the ciliated columnar cells, and the mucus itself all protect the body by establishing a defense system in the upper airway, or the nose and the sinuses.

A base layer below the goblet cells and the ciliated columnar cells is formed by basal cells. These cells form the barrier preventing infection and toxins from entering the body through the sinuses. The basal lining is a defense shield for the body in the same way that your skin protects your insides from foreign substances.

WHERE MUCUS GOES: THE OSTIOMEATAL COMPLEX

The ciliated cells move the mucus over the sinus membranes in a specific direction, so that the mucous blanket with its trapped particles can be excreted. These cells each contain between 50 and 200 tiny microscopic hairs called cilia, which move at an astounding rate of close to 800 times a minute. These cilia cells beat like a sweeping broom, pushing the mucus through each of the sinuses from the front of the nose to the back. The back of the nose is called the nasopharynx, because this area connects the nose and the throat (pharynx).

You might think that gravity is pulling the mucus along. However, this is not always the case. For example, the hair cells in the maxillary sinus lift the mucus with its trapped particles along its side walls against gravity. And the hair cells in the frontal sinus sweep in a specific direction as well. The maxillary sinus drains its mucus through an opening located at the top of the sinus, and then into an area called the infundibulum. The infundibulum is part of the ostiomeatal complex (OMC), which includes the anterior ethmoid sinuses (Diagram 7). The OMC is called "the key to the sinuses" because the frontal sinus, the maxillary sinus, and the anterior ethmoid sinuses drain into this area.

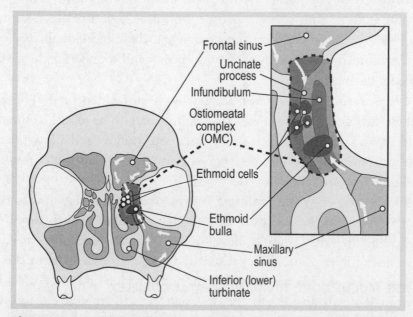

Diagram 7 The Ostiomeatal Complex is called "the key to the sinuses" because the frontal sinus, the maxillary sinus, and the anterior ethmoid sinuses drain into this area.

When the OMC gets blocked or plugged up, the anterior ethmoids and the frontal and maxillary sinuses have nowhere to drain. The mucous blanket then backs up into the frontal and maxillary sinuses, and these areas become inflamed.

OUT OF THE NOSE AND INTO THE THROAT: THE NASOPHARYNX

The mucus, now carrying the trapped dirt and other unwanted particles, leaves the nose and is moved into the nasopharynx, the passageway located above the soft part of the roof of the mouth, or the soft palate. The nasopharynx connects the ears and nose to the throat. The bottom of the nasal cavity itself is formed by the roof of the hard palate and a portion of the soft palate. The soft palate moves when we swallow, covering up the velopharyngeal opening (the opening between the soft palate and the back of the throat), which connects the nasopharynx to the pharynx, or throat (Diagram 8). It is this closure that prevents food from regurgitating into your nose when you swallow. When this opening is compromised, as in people who have a cleft palate, it cannot close, and food is forced into the nose when these individuals swallow. Furthermore, they have difficulty with speech and sound as if they were speaking through their nose.

On each side of the nasopharynx lies a eustachian tube. The eustachian tubes connect your ears (the middle ears, to be exact) to the nasopharynx. These tubes open every time you swallow and allow for the equalization of air pressure between the middle ear and the constantly changing pressure in the outside world.

In the case of young children, mucus drains from the sinuses into the nasopharynx, passing over the eustachian tubes. These tubes are small, and when they begin to develop they're fairly horizontal, making them susceptible to infection caused by backed up mucus from the sinuses into the ears. As we get older, the tubes widen and the eustachian tubes angle downward, easing the drainage from the middle ear into the nasopharynx (Diagram 9).

The adenoid bed, another common spot for infection, is also located in the back of the nasopharynx. Like the tonsils, the adenoid bed is

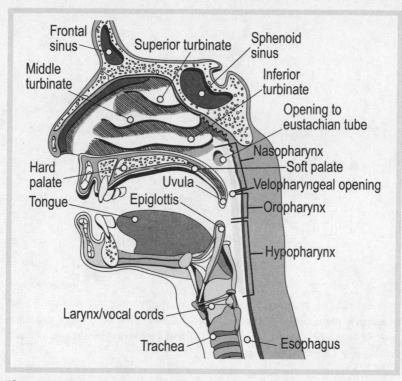

Diagram 8 A side view of the sinuses and the nasopharynx.

made up of lymphoid tissue that guards the throat from infection. Together, the adenoid bed, tonsils, and other small lymphoid glands in the throat form a ring of protective tissue called Waldeyer's ring, which defends against infection and cancer. We each have many sets of tonsils, or tonsillar tissue. There are tonsils in the base of the tongue called the lingual (tongue) tonsils and tonsils in the sides of the back of the throat, called the palatine tonsils. The palatine tonsils are the ones that are taken out in children who suffer from tonsillitis. The adenoid bed typically disappears by the age of 5 or 6. However, in children with considerable infection, the adenoid bed swells and may obstruct the eustachian tubes and possibly the nose and the sinuses as well. Rarely are the adenoids present or swollen in adults, although I have seen cases in which they were present in patients with severe chronic infection.

The mucus then passes into the back of the throat, which is home to yet another set of mucus-producing glands. These glands, along with

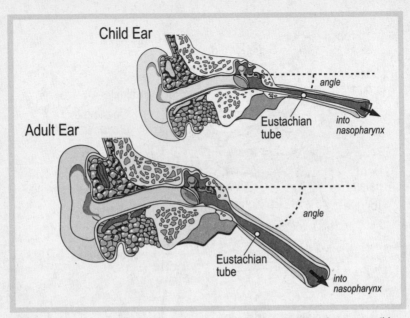

Diagram 9 The eustachian tubes are horizontal in a child's ear, making them susceptible to infection. In an adult's ear, the tubes are angled downward, easing the drainage of mucus from the inner ear into the nasopharynx.

the salivary and mucus glands of the mouth, create the slippery surface that assists us when we swallow food.

The Ear

As I already noted, the ear is connected to the sinuses through the eustachian tube. When the sinuses are inflamed, the eustachian tubes also become inflamed. Infections in the sinuses can pass into the ears through these tubes. Primary ear problems—such as recurrent ear infections, benign tumors, pain, noise, tinnitus, and dizziness—may be caused by sinus and nasal problems.

The ear is made up of three parts: the outer (external) ear, the middle ear, and the inner ear (Diagram 10). Each part serves a particular function. The external ear is the part of the ear that you can see. It extends into the ear canal, which connects the outside world with the eardrum.

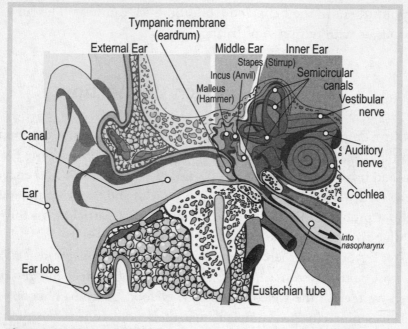

Diagram 10 The anatomy of the ear.

The external ear is covered with skin, which protects the external ear from infection, most notably swimmer's ear. The external ear also produces cerumen, otherwise known as earwax. Regardless of what any well-intentioned parent might have told you, the external ear continuously removes the cerumen by itself, without your needing to use cotton swabs. And cerumen is actually good: It aids in fighting infection in the external ear.

The middle ear is the area behind the eardrum. You really can't see the middle ear, but your doctor can determine if it is infected by the presence of fluid that he or she can see through the eardrum. As sound hits the eardrum, it moves three little bones in the middle ear—the malleus (hammer), the incus (anvil), and the stapes (stirrup)—to create a fluid wave into the inner ear.

The inner ear is made up of the cochlea, which is shaped like a snail, and the labyrinth, which is composed of three semicircular canals. The inner ear can't be seen because it is encased in the temporal bone of the skull. The cochlea sends signals to the auditory nerve, which transmits them to the brain and—prestol!—we can hear. The labyrinth also aids us with our sense of balance.

The Nose-Stomach Connection

After passing through the nasopharynx, mucus is swallowed, dropping into the throat (pharynx) and behind the voice box through the esophagus and finally into the stomach (Diagram 11). The acids and enzymes in the stomach kill bacteria, viruses, and molds and break up the mucus without problems. Finally, the mucus and its dirt particles pass through the digestive tract, get destroyed, and are finally excreted.

Yet beyond this, there are many other direct connections between the nose and the stomach. For instance, we often feel hunger pains when we receive the welcoming smells of food. Also, many people, especially senior citizens, complain that their nose runs when they eat. You may have experienced this yourself when you eat hot soup or spicy

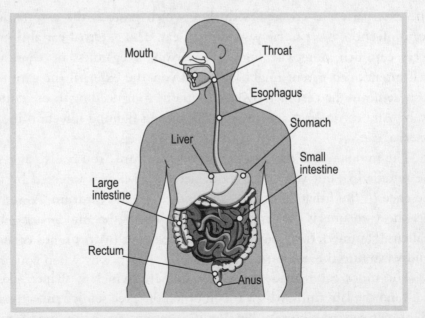

Diagram 11 Mucus follows the same path as food, traveling through the esophagus and into the stomach, where it is broken down.

foods. I believe that this connection involves the autonomic nervous system, a very complex system of nerves that connects our entire body and is responsible for seemingly involuntary bodily functions. The autonomic nervous system prepares and organizes the set of events that occur from the time that we feel hungry (i.e., when our blood sugars drop) and smell food to the time that our food is ingested and processed, providing nutrients to our body. For example, eating triggers a response in the nose that can cause congestion.

Our Bodies, Our Nose

Beyond mere breathing and mucus production, the nose is integrally connected to the functioning of the rest of the body. One important factor is our sense of smell. The cribriform plate lies at the top of the inside of the nose, which is the area under the brain near the middle, superior, and supreme turbinates and the septum. Tiny perforations in this plate transmit the sense of smell to the brain by way of the olfactory nerve. Anything that has a smell releases a chemical, called an odorant, through the process of evaporation. This odorant is picked up by an olfactory nerve ending, called a receptor cell. There are 10–20 million receptor cells in each nasal chamber lining the cribriform plate and nose. These receptors fire off an impulse in the nerve, which is sent to the nerve's olfactory bulb. The olfactory bulb contains receptors called sensory nerve cells that transmit the information about the odors to the brain. The brain matches the information to memories of earlier received smells. This gives us our sense of smell.

Our sense of smell is very important and often taken for granted. It helps us experience pleasure by allowing us to encounter good smells and to taste our food. Approximately 80 percent of our sense of taste comes from decoding the fragrance of food. This is why when you have a stuffy nose, food doesn't seem to have much flavor.

Furthermore, our sense of smell is integral in picking a mate. Every person has a unique odor. This odor becomes very important in the selection process of choosing friends, especially a mate, just as we are

attracted to the way others look and sound. The multibillion-dollar perfume and fragrance industry capitalizes on this human connection by
creating scents that we find attractive in perfumes, colognes, soaps, powders, and deodorants.

In addition, the nasal septum houses a structure called the vomerine
gland. This gland can detect pheromones, complex chemicals released
by the body that create a unique, yet subtle scent. Pheromones are believed to be partially responsible for providing the brain with information used when choosing a mate. There has been much controversy
about pheromones in recent years, because many fragrance producers
claim that they place such chemicals in their perfumes and colognes.

Some scientists believe that the sense of smell also has a role in the
act of sex itself. For many people, the sense of smell is important in the
arousal period leading up to intercourse. It is also one reason why some
people may not fully experience the range of sexual satisfaction when
their nose is congested.

The Nose and Lungs

The nose is the upper most structure of the respiratory system and can
be thought of as the portal to the lungs. Air can enter the body only
through the nose or the mouth. In a healthy person, the majority of air
enters through the nose (except in times of exertion or distress). Newborn babies breathe exclusively through the nose. If their nose is partially obstructed, they will not be able to feed well and will have
difficulty breathing. If the nose of a newborn is totally obstructed he or
she won't be able to breathe at all. A newborn's voice box essentially
protrudes into the nasopharynx, cutting off the mouth from the airway.
A newborn with a total obstruction of the nose will have a bluish skin
tone and will need the instillation of a special breathing tube.

As children get older, they are able to breathe through their mouth
more readily because their voice box drops as they grow, permitting the
air that enters their mouth to flow into the lungs (Diagram 12). Adults
automatically breathe through their nose with a closed mouth, unless

they experience nasal blockage, which forces them to breathe through an open mouth. Most people have partial obstruction of their nose and breathe through their nose and their mouth. This is not normal, even though many of us think that it is, because we are designed to breathe through our nose only.

Once air has been taken in through the nose, it passes along the same path as the mucus: it first moves into the sinuses and gets filtered. It then comes out of the sinuses and enters the nasopharynx and the throat. At this point, air and mucus take different paths. The mucus passes behind the larynx into the esophagus, while the air passes through the larynx and into the trachea (the windpipe), the bronchi, and lungs. Once air reaches the lung tissue, the air passes into the bronchioles, which are small branches, and then the alveoli, which are the terminal ends of the airway. It is in the alveoli that oxygen passes through the membranes of the lung into the venous bloodstream (Diagram 13).

In the bloodstream, oxygen links up with red blood cells that travel through pulmonary veins and blood vessels toward the heart. The heart

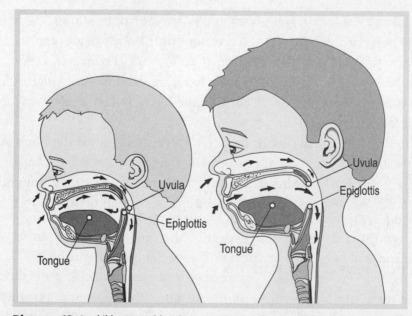

Diagram 12 As children get older, their voice boxes drop, permitting the air that enters their mouth to flow into the lungs.

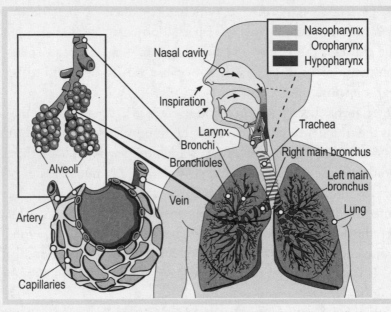

	Nasopharynx
	Oropharynx
	Hypopharynx

Nasal cavity

Inspiration

Larynx
Bronchi
Bronchioles

Trachea

Right main bronchus

Left main bronchus

Lung

Alveoli

Vein

Artery

Capillaries

Diagram 13 When air reaches the alveoli in the lungs, oxygen passes through the membranes of the lung into the venous bloodstream.

then distributes the oxygen-rich blood to your organs, muscles, brain, other parts of the body via the arteries. Your body's tissues replace the oxygen (O_2) with carbon dioxide (CO_2). After the arterial blood releases the oxygen, the veins take the deoxygenated blood (which is low in oxygen and high in CO_2) back to the heart, which sends it to lungs to pick up more oxygen.

If the nose doesn't work properly, the air taken into the lungs will not be filtered, humidified, and heated. This decreases the exchange of oxygen with carbon dioxide in the bloodstream, and cells throughout the body will not get the proper amount of oxygen delivered to them (Diagram 14).

THE HORMONE CONNECTION

Many pregnant women experience swelling. While they might notice that their trunk, limbs, and face swell, they might not realize that when their outside swells their inside swells as well. This includes the inside of

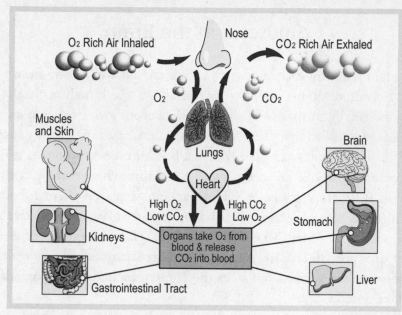

Diagram 14 Oxygen is delivered into the bloodstream from the lungs. The oxygen-rich blood then travels to other parts of the body.

their nose and sinus membranes. Approximately 30 percent of pregnant women report experiencing nasal congestion, usually during the end of the first trimester.

Increases in estrogen levels during the monthly menstrual cycle can also induce nasal swelling and enhance mucus production. Conversely, when women enter menopause they tend to experience a drop in their estrogen levels, and the amount and quality of their mucus changes. As a result, these women also complain about more nasal congestion.

ADRENALINE

When you are intensely exercising or experiencing anxiety, your body sets off an instinctual "flight or fright response." When this occurs, adrenaline is released, which causes your nasal and sinus membranes to shrink. This allows you to breathe easier, so that more air can get into your lungs, and your body will have the additional oxygen it requires.

Sinuses and the Brain

The brain relies on the sinuses in various ways as well. Aside from providing clean, oxygen-rich air to the brain via the bloodstream, the sinuses aid the brain in several autonomic nervous system responses. For instance, we know that there is a nasopulmonary reflex that causes a drop in oxygen saturation levels throughout the body when your nose and/or nasopharynx are obstructed. I see this when there is a tissue mass in the nasopharynx or when packing is placed there to stop a nosebleed. A second reflex occurs when you are splashed in the face and nose with cold water: You stop breathing. The sinuses and nose also affect and are affected by the complex structure of the autonomic nervous system, which comprises the parasympathetic and sympathetic nervous systems.

Identifying a Problem

Now that you understand how your entire body is connected to your nose, you can imagine what a healthy respiratory system feels like. When everything is working properly, you should feel alert most of the time. Air should flow freely through your nose to your lungs and you should be able to breathe easily. Mucus should not obstruct your nose, affect your throat, or cause your stomach to act up. At night, you should be able to sleep soundly, unaffected by snoring or restlessness. When you wake up, you should feel refreshed and ready to face another day.

Yet for all the body's intricate and perfect anatomical structuring, many things can, and often do, go wrong. When the nose and sinuses don't function as they were intended, the rest of the body suffers. If you feel that your breathing is compromised in any way, day or night, you are probably experiencing a nasal or sinus problem. The good news is that there are effective and permanent treatments for your symptoms and conditions. No matter how awful you feel today, you can feel better by following the suggestions outlined in this book. You can be treated, either naturally, with medication, or with surgery, depending on the severity of your condition. The knowledge that you have obtained in this chapter will allow you to understand the different treatment options better and will help you make informed decisions as you make your way back to health.

CHAPTER 2

THE SYMPTOMS OF CHRONIC AIRWAY-DIGESTIVE INFLAMMATORY DISEASE

The Sinus Revolution begins when we recognize that even the slightest, seemingly most insignificant symptom should be taken seriously. The human body is made to function at an optimal level. That means that with good health, you should not have any aches or pains. You should smell odors clearly, and breathe through your nose comfortably. However, if any part of your body is not functioning optimally, then you are suffering from some sort of complication.

Many people live with symptoms, yet do not recognize them. They think that they are normal or are experiencing the trials of aging. And while these seemingly inconsequential symptoms may not cause significant pain now, it's not the way your body was meant to run. Over time, a small inconvenience can easily turn into a larger, more significant health problem.

The first step then is to recognize the symptoms most commonly associated with the nose and the sinuses. When any of these symptoms appear, it is a sign that something in this pathway has gone wrong and can—and should—be corrected.

When Your Sinuses Fail

Sinus problems begin when the sinus pathways become obstructed as a result of inflammation, which causes the nasal membranes to swell, narrowing the air's pathway. Inflammation in the breathing system occurs when you are exposed to an infection (stemming from bacteria, a virus, or mold), allergens, or other irritants (such as pollution, cigarette smoke, car exhaust, or perfumes).

Many of these substances are in the air all the time, yet some people are more affected by them than others. The inflammatory cycle is triggered by these and other irritants when they are coupled with a genetic predisposition, causing certain people to react. For instance, why are some people sensitive to cigarette smoke while others are not bothered by it? Why are some people sensitive to specific allergens, and others not? Why do some people develop an infection, while others are equally exposed, but not affected?

The answers are still not known. But what we do know is that these phenomena are determined by the genetic makeup of each person. And, although research in human genetics has made great strides, there is still much about individual differences in our immune system that we don't understand. So currently, we have to treat these phenomena, and the related symptoms and conditions on a case-by-case basis.

Your airway can also be compromised because of your unique anatomical structure. Sinus and nasal narrowing can occur if you were born with a physical defect within the nose. For example, the nasal cavity can be narrowed by a deviated septum or sinuses that never developed properly. Just as some people are short and others tall, some small and others large, the sinus pathways among individuals also vary. The passageways may be intrinsically narrow or small. Often, the turbinates can develop with an air cell within them, or they may be large or positioned in the middle of the airway. In the worst case, rare tumors like papilloma (nasal or sinus warts) or cancer can cause blockage of the nose or sinuses. Any of these anomalies can prevent air from optimally passing through the nose and sinuses.

Trauma, or a blow to the head, can also cause a narrowing of the passageways. A fall taken at a young age could have caused your septum to deviate, growing along a crooked line as you developed. You might have even fractured your nose on your way out of the birth canal, and you may not even know that it was traumatized. On the other hand, you may be acutely aware of a nose injury, such as getting elbowed playing sports. No matter what the initial cause or when the air pathway was altered, the air currently passing through your nose circulates with abnormal motion that can cause erosion of the membranes, leading to drying, crusting, and/or scabbing. It can even lead to bleeding as the erosion becomes more significant. Polyps, which are benign growths or tumors, can form within the nose and sinus cavities from any of the irritants that cause inflammation. Some scientists believe that any inflammation in the nasal passages leads to swelling and then to infection, which ultimately causes polyp formation.

Once the cycle of inflammation begins, it is very difficult to correct it. The initial inflammation leads to obstruction. As this obstruction worsens, it causes more inflammation around the obstructed area. This causes stagnation of the mucus and crusting and/or scabbing, all which create an ideal breeding ground for bacteria and molds to grow. This growth of infection causes more inflammation and swelling and more obstruction. Ultimately, both inflammation and blockage create a cycle that worsens with every breath you take.

Caustic agents like chemicals, pollution and/or smoking can also damage the normal movement of the ciliated hair cells—for example, smoking can cause these hair cells to become singed from the heat of the ingested cigarette. Nicotine also causes the nose's blood vessels to constrict to the point that the hair cells can become damaged or paralyzed. Metals that are present in air pollution from car exhaust or chemicals in new carpeting can damage the cilia as well. As a result, the sinuses stop draining properly: The mucus backup exacerbates and worsens the inflammation and the obstruction, all making the initial infection worse. This cycle will continue to get worse until it is broken.

Meanwhile, your normal mucus production has also changed. What was once clear running fluid is now thick and static. There is also a change in its acidity (pH). Ironically, the body's natural reaction to airway inflammation is to produce more mucus to wash the inflammation and infection away. This mucus continues to pool and starts to thicken as its water content evaporates. This is worsened when your body raises its temperature to fight off the infection. At this point, the body's defenses start to release white blood cells into the mucus to fight the bacteria, viruses, or molds, all of which can further change the pH and consistency. The white blood cells release toxic substances and enzymes to kill the infection. Some of these cells start "eating" the infection to kill it, a process called phagocytosis. These toxic substances cause damage to the cilia, more inflammation and swelling, and chronically can cause thickening of the membranes. As each sinus cavity closes due to swelling, the oxygen in the cavity itself decreases, making each of these closed cavities more prone to infection. All of this leads to sinus disease, and ultimately to chronic airway-digestive inflammatory disease (CAID) (Diagram 15).

Chronic problems occur when there are breaks in the nasal membranes that should be keeping infection out of the body. When these membranes are broken, an infection can enter the body. Bacteria pass

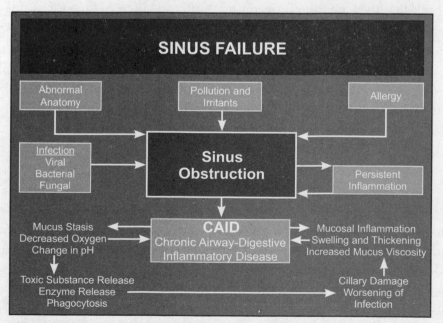

Diagram 15 There are many different factors that lead to CAID.

into the bloodstream, and when their levels are sufficient, your body re-acts again by raising its temperature to kill the infection. This rise in body temperature can occur for short periods of time as a result of spik-ing bacteria levels in the bloodstream or may occur over longer periods of time when the infection is bad enough to cause a higher, more con-stant level of bacteria. The fever may be low grade as a result of expo-sure to constant chronic infection or it may be higher in reaction to an acute infection, or a sudden high exposure to bacteria.

I FEEL MISERABLE

At this point you are not feeling well at all. Your nose is stuffed, and you may have a headache. You may feel rundown and your thinking is clouded. But because you can still mostly function, you continue to go about your days and nights not feeling well but not really complaining either. You may have felt this way so often or for so long that you have come to think that this is acceptable or even normal. But it is not.

Often people relay that their family members or significant other think that they are just complaining. Sufferers often tell me that some-one will say to them, "It's just a cold, get over it," or "What's the big deal? It's a stuffy nose." For many people, this is probably correct: When our sinuses fail for a brief period, it can be caused by a cold that will quickly pass. But for others, their sinuses cause them to feel sick all of the time. In fact, it can be debilitating.

CAID

In the past, your sinus condition would be diagnosed depending on where your doctor believed the majority of the inflammation first occurred. For example, I used to consider the nose and the sinuses as separate entities. I spoke about rhinitis when I was dealing with an in-flammation of the nose, and sinusitis when I referred to inflammation of the sinuses. While it is possible to suffer from each of these entities separately, we now realize that inflammation of the sinuses invariably affects the nose. So we now refer to inflammation of the nose and sinuses together as chronic rhinosinusitis (CRS).

Doctors also believed that sinus problems stopped at the nose. But we now know our individual parts are intricately connected, and what affects the sinuses ultimately affects how the entire body functions. Once sinus problems begin, they spark a chain reaction throughout the body. For example, we know that when the sinuses fail, the air that is breathed into the lungs can become contaminated, which can damage the membranes of the lungs. The lungs can respond by constricting, as is the case with asthma—if you suffer from this, you may feel tight in your chest and hear a wheezing sound as you breath. The oxygen supply to the bloodstream then becomes compromised, and the entire body can experience a loss of oxygen. We now believe that the inflammatory process affecting the nose, the sinuses, and the lungs is one and the same process. This revolutionary thinking now allows us to treat the problems of sinusitis, allergy, and asthma together as one. The result is that my patients are feeling better.

You may have been told that you constantly feel sick because you are suffering from allergies. While your allergies might have been treated, your sinuses were largely ignored; consequently, you continue to feel sick, even though you are taking your allergy medication. Or you may have been told that you had sinus disease, but your asthma was not treated. Or you were treated for asthma but not for your sinus problems. In each of these cases, you were given only part of the diagnosis.

Luckily, those days of misdiagnoses are over. We now believe that while the initial cause of sinus inflammation may vary, inflammation can affect the entire or different select parts of the respiratory tree from the tip of the nose to the smallest end branches of the lung. This thinking intricately connects the conditions of allergies and asthma to the workings, or malfunctions, of the sinuses. Ultimately, inflammation is what causes us to feel sick from any of these disease processes: sinus disease, allergies, or asthma. Therefore, the disease processes that affect the nose, sinuses, and lungs are simply different limbs of the same disease. I like to call this inflammation chronic airway inflammation (CAI).

CAI can affect the entire airway as well as the upper and lower gastrointestinal (GI) tract. Just as the nose is anatomically connected to the gastrointestinal tract through the mucous passageway, infected mucus will drip down the esophagus and into the stomach and enter the GI tract. It upsets the balance of bacteria, which can cause the stomach to react and create acid. The stomach and the esophagus meet at the gastroesophageal junction, which is near the diaphragm, the muscle that controls your breathing. Muscle fibers wrap around this junction and form a closure that is intended to prevent the stomach contents from backing up. If this junction becomes weak, or if the stomach bulges through this junction (called a hiatal hernia) then it becomes easier for the contents of the stomach to back up into the esophagus, causing reflux. The reflux contains acid, and if the acid stays in contact with the membranes of the esophagus long enough it can burn the membranes. This is what gives you a feeling of fullness in your chest, burning, heartburn, or indigestion, and it is called gastroesophageal reflux disease (GERD). If the acids do not stay long enough within the esophagus but instead continue to reflux up to the larynx (voice box), pharynx (throat), and drip into the airway, this is called laryngopharyngeal reflux disease (LPRD). The acids may even reflux into the nasopharynx and/or nose and sinuses.

If the acids reach as high as the larynx (voice box), they can cause swelling, which can result in soreness, hoarseness, or the feeling that something is caught in your throat. The acid can then drop into the trachea and the small airways of the lungs, causing further inflammation, setting off an asthma attack or causing a chemical tracheitis, bronchitis, or even pneumonia. It can cause the larynx to spasm: When this occurs, the larynx closes to prevent further aspiration of stomach contents into the lung, and you feel like you can't breathe for a few seconds. This is called laryngospasm.

CAI is often connected to various stomach ailments that cause reflux. As well, patients with these disease processes can suffer from snoring and/or sleep apnea. Therefore, I refer to CAI, LPRD/GERD, and snoring/sleep apnea collectively, calling this disease chronic airway-digestive inflammatory disease. Furthermore, some believe that the airway inflammatory processes are connected to all of the inflammatory diseases of the gut, including Crohn's disease and ulcerative colitis. At this time, there is not enough conclusive evidence; however, it appears that many people with digestive ailments also suffer from sinus disease.

From Head to Toe: Signs and Symptoms of and Conditions Related to CAID

Many people go through life without their sinuses functioning properly. Those of us who suffer from CAID may experience only minor problems; but for others, life can be miserable. Some sufferers have mild symptoms or have a gradually worsening condition, so they think they are well when they actually are not. These people are usually bothered only when they have an acute flare-up.

Worse, they may believe that their chronic symptoms are normal and accept them as a part of life. For example, some people tell me that they frequently expel "normal" yellow-green mucus. Yet, yellow-green mucus is not normal at all! Others tell me that they can never breathe through their nose and always breathe through their mouth, thinking that all people breathe in this manner. I've even met people who have told me that they have had "a cold" for over a year! There are others who are frequently bothered by a consistent set of symptoms, which they may find annoying but not quite debilitating. Some seek treatment, whereas others just live with it.

In another scenario, you may have a symptom that may cause further damage or long-term disability and you don't even know it. For example, sleep apnea, which is also part of CAID, is directly linked to heart disease. Sleep apnea alone is responsible for many heart attacks and strokes. If you don't recognize the signs and symptoms of sleep apnea and treat it now, it can disastrously affect you later on in life. And even though the snoring with sleep apnea doesn't cause pain or discomfort, except maybe the constant badgering of a significant other who cannot sleep, the fact is that sleep apnea is called a "silent" killer. By understanding and treating these conditions now, you can avoid the more considerable long-term problems that are more difficult to address later.

On the other end of the spectrum are people who recognize that they are sick all the time. There are those who become so debilitated from their sinus problems that they can't function. Many of these people go from doctor to doctor and are unable to find relief. They often

Signs Versus Symptoms

There is a significant difference between a sign and a symptom. A *sign* is objective evidence (something that can be measured) or an objective manifestation of a disease or disorder. A *symptom*, on the other hand, is a subjective perceptible change in the body or its functions as it pertains to a disease or disorder. For example, when you have a fever, you may complain of feeling warm. This feeling is considered as a symptom, because it is subjective. But when you take your temperature, the measurement is an objective sign. Therefore, your temperature of 99.7°F (a sign) and your feeling warm (a symptom) are characteristics of an illness. Every disease, including CAID, has identifying signs and symptoms.

suffer from symptoms ranging from chronic fatigue to debilitating headaches. Others can't breathe at night, and as a result have difficulty sleeping. Others tell me that their spouse or partner complains of their incessant snoring. Others have night sweats, chills, or a low-grade fever. CAID causes a variety of easily recognizable signs and symptoms. You may be experiencing a combination of these signs or symptoms or only one. Your experience with each particular symptom may range from mild to severe, yet the underlying cause is the same: inflammation.

IDENTIFYING CAID

The first step in improving your health is to identify the signs and symptoms you may be experiencing. Sometimes, a particular symptom may represent the actual diagnosis, such as when a patient comes in and tells me that every time she is near fresh-cut grass she begins to sneeze. This reaction is a common symptom of an allergy to grass. Or an individual symptom may represent just part of the diagnosis, especially if there are multiple problems occurring at the same time.

It is, therefore, important for you to first understand the definition of each of the symptoms. As you start to speak the same language as your physician, it will make it easier for you to organize your thoughts and report your story accurately. Every doctor's main role is to organize your experience into the proper diagnosis or diagnoses. I always tell my patients that without their help, I don't have a chance at helping them feel better. If you can become a good detective and accurately relay your symptoms to your physician, then he or she will be able to make a more accurate diagnosis.

Read through each of the following descriptions and see if you can identify whether you are currently experiencing that sign or symptom. You may have had some of the symptoms in the past or may have never noticed others. Read all the descriptions so you'll be able to recognize the conditions if they ever occur. If you are regularly suffering from any of the symptoms, you may be diagnosed with CAID. Because the primary branches of CAID have overlapping symptoms, it is first important to identify how your body is feeling. Later, I will explain how you can identify which branch of CAID you are suffering from and provide the appropriate treatment for your symptoms.

Remember, each of the conditions discussed in the following sections should not be considered as a "normal" state for healthy people. Many of these symptoms, like partial nasal blockage or snoring, may be misconstrued as normal because they are not life threatening, or causing acute pain. Even something that makes you chronically uncomfortable should be dealt with: You do not need to learn to live with any sort of discomfort. All of these symptoms can be treated, and they will, in time, disappear.

SIGNS AND SYMPTOMS OF A SINUS INFECTION

Nasal Discharge
When inflammation affects the nose and/or the sinuses, your nose will run, because the nose and sinuses will produce additional mucus to try to wash away the offending agent whether infection, allergy or irritating particle like smoke, car exhaust, or pollution. An increase in nasal discharge can make you feel like you have to continually wipe your nose, or it can increase the amount of normal postnasal drip and make you feel like you are drowning in mucus or choking. It can also make you feel so stuffy that you need to clear your nose.

The nasal discharge is clear if you have a viral infection or you experience an allergic flare-up; however, when bacteria cause the inflammation, the mucus will become discolored. It can be milky white, yellow, green, brown, or any mixture. If mold is causing the inflammation, the mucus will most often be discolored with black, white, or green particles, similar to the mold that grows on bread, cheese, or fruit. Fungi can also look like axle grease.

Inflamed sinuses produce mucus that is different from normal mucus. Whatever the color, infected mucus is thick and sticky; often its consistency can be described as gelatinous. The pH of the mucus also changes, becoming more acidic. This occurs as a result of the substances that are released to fight infection, reduce inflammation, and/or react to allergens. The mucus can also look and feel like the jelly that is found around refrigerated fish, or it can look like apricot jelly or egg drop soup. It can also feel like rubber cement glue, or axle grease.

Nasal Obstruction/Nasal Congestion

As a result of inflammation, nasal stuffiness and nasal obstruction or blockage can occur. You might not notice the almost complete nasal blockage, because the body's natural tendency is to compensate for this obstruction through mouth breathing. Because this occurs over a long period of time, you might not even recognize that you are breathing through your mouth.

When you feel that your nose has become stuffy, you may be experiencing one of two reactions. The first is the actual swelling caused by the inflammatory nature of the nasal membranes. The second is caused by the thickened mucus itself, which leads to further obstruction. The thickened mucus makes it is hard to breathe because of the blockage that it causes.

Significant nasal congestion is uncomfortable and annoying. It is also a common symptom for those with low thyroid levels or diabetes. This is just another example why you should not take any of these symptoms lightly. If you are chronically congested, all year long, see your doctor to exclude these serious diseases from your overall diagnosis.

Headaches

When the sinuses become obstructed, pressure gradients are created between the closed sinus and the changing air pressure in the environment.

This can cause headaches that range from dull pressure to piercing pain. Sinus membranes are very sensitive to changes in pressure, causing you to feel a significant amount of pain with even a small pressure differential. When the pressure of the world outside the nose is less than the pressure in the obstructed sinus cell then the air in the sinuses expands, applying pressure to the walls of the sinus. Conversely, when the pressure outside the sinus is more than the pressure inside, the pressure in the sinus becomes negative and tugs on the sinus wall, pulling the membrane away from the bony wall. These forces can also cause direct pressure and inflammation on the nerves passing through the sinuses, causing neuralgia, a considerably painful condition. While a deviated septum itself cannot cause headaches, a deviated septum that applies pressure on another part of the nose can be a source of headache pain.

Ear Squeeze

When there are significant pressure changes in the environment and your sinuses are obstructed, you can develop a pain in the face or forehead that feels like a sharp stab, as if you were being attacked with a knife. This pain can be accompanied by a nose bleed: The negative pressure can tear a blood vessel or the membrane itself. This is called "sinus squeeze" because it feels as if someone were putting your sinuses into a vice and squeezing it hard enough to cause pain. Sinus squeeze most often occurs when scuba diving or sky flying in an airplane because of the great fluctuations in air pressure. However, it can also occur when you are driving or riding on a train through a mountainous area.

You may also experience this same sharp pain in your ear. Ear squeeze occurs when there is a closure of the eustachian tube(s), combined with pressure changes in the environment. The eustachian tubes allow us to equalize the pressure in our ears. We all swallow 12–15 times a minute. Each time we swallow, the eustachian tube opens up to equalize the pressure in the middle ear. When this no longer occurs properly, the ears develop pressure gradients. This can be exacerbated when you climb a mountain, fly in an airplane, ride an elevator in a tall building, or scuba or sky dive. This is the reason that you may experience difficulty popping your ears when you fly.

The pressure can get so severe that it can tear a vessel in the eardrum, causing bleeding into the eardrum or middle ear, or the blood can run from the ear canal itself. Although rare, you may experience temporary or long-term hearing loss, tinnitus (a ringing in your ear), or dizziness (vertigo, or spinning or loss of balance), if the trauma from the pressure change is severe enough. These symptoms can most likely be reversed if treated immediately, so it is important for you to see an oto-laryngologist (an ear, nose, and throat (ENT) physician) who is experienced with this type of problem.

Postnasal Drip

Everyone produces 1–2 liters of mucus each day. Most of the time you swallow it unnoticed. However, when mucus is particularly thick or excessive, you will notice it. You might feel as if you were choking or that something were caught in your throat. This feeling is referred to as postnasal drip. The acidic pH of the mucus is itself inflammatory and can also cause a sore or scratchy throat.

Sneezing

When dust or other particles enter your nose, your body's protective response is to sneeze to expel the particle. That is why when people suffer from allergies, they sneeze a lot. When allergens land on the membranes of the nose, and the normal reaction is to sneeze to expel the allergens.

Cough

Mucus usually passes down the throat to the esophagus. If it instead lands on the vocal cords, it can pass into the windpipe and then into the lungs. When this occurs, your body will rely on another protective mechanism: You will start coughing so that the mucus does not continue to travel along this path. You cough to expel the mucus from the airways. We often think that coughing is bad; although coughing can be irritating, coughing is really necessary to defend your lungs against infection.

However, constant or chronic coughing is a symptom that must be dealt with because it can lead to other, more significant problems. For example, women often report that incontinence accompanies bouts of coughing. Chronic cough is defined as a cough lasting over 3 weeks. Chronic cough is not contagious. Many who suffer from chronic cough can't sleep, and their significant others are awakened by their coughing fits. Even today, there is no single test that will determine what is causing a chronic cough. Instead, most doctors will have you go through a systematic elimination of probable causes. We know that the most common causes for chronic cough include those related to CAID: asthma, postnasal drip, chronic rhinosinusitis, LPRD and/or GERD. In a recent Mayo Clinic study, researchers found that more than one third of chronic cough patients were also experiencing an inflammation of the sinuses. It now seems that underlying sinus inflammation should be considered as a major cause of chronic cough.

Yet CAID, and even sinusitis alone, is often overlooked by physicians as a culprit in chronic cough. The high percentage of sinus inflammation in patients with cough in the Mayo Clinic study suggests that those individuals should be seen by an otolaryngologist, who specializes in sinus problems and cough. Yet many people with chronic cough are instead treated by their primary-care physician (internist, family physician, or pediatrician) or a pulmonologist (lung specialist). Unfortunately, these physicians typically never address the sinus problem that is causing the cough, and these patients never get better.

In addition, many have been told by their physicians to learn to live with their coughs. Worse, they have been mistakenly diagnosed as having a nervous cough, which means that their coughs are triggered by being in an uncomfortable situation. I do not believe that there is such a condition as a nervous cough, and there is no diagnosis code for nervous cough in the *International Classification of Diseases*, the reference book all physicians use to classify a diagnosis. In my mind, this diagnosis is made when the physician can't figure out what is causing a cough.

Chronic cough can have adverse social, psychological, or physical effects. I always tell the families of my patients that even if the cough is disturbing to them, they need to have some empathy because most people who suffer from a chronic cough just want to jump out of their own skin. In another Mayo Clinic survey, researchers found that chronic cough patients reported significant social and emotional problems. They were frustrated, irritable, and angry over the ineffectiveness of therapies. They felt helplessness, which had a profound effect on their quality of life. Many people are debilitated by their cough. They report that their friends and family do not want to be around them because their cough is so disturbing or because they fear the spread of infection.

Throat Clearing

When infected mucus drips or gets caught in the back of your throat it can cause discomfort. You will naturally try to get rid of the feeling by employing another protective mechanism: clearing your throat. Throat clearing is related to coughing but is different in that it is a reaction to mucus in the throat, not in the lungs. Furthermore, because it is sometimes hard to dislodge the thick mucus, you may continue to have the dripping sensation even after you attempt to clear your throat. Many of my patients who suffer from this problem tell me that they will not go out socially because they are embarrassed by their frequent throat clearing.

Even during an office examination, some physicians are not able to see the mucus in the back of the throat. Usually, they are not looking deep enough. These physicians may misdiagnose their patients with GERD or LPRD (which can also cause throat clearing). Worse, a physician may tell his or her patients that throat clearing is a "nervous habit."

I have suffered from this symptom, and I know that it is a very irritating and very real physiological condition. I have been told by some of my ENT colleagues that my incessant throat clearing is not a physiological problem but rather a nervous tic. When I showed them how to properly suction out the mucus that was dripping from my sinuses to the back of my throat, my throat clearing stopped. They could not believe the amount of mucus that was present in my sinuses, which they could not see on general inspection. Furthermore, when I suffer from excessive mucus production, my GERD and LPRD start to act up, which makes my throat clearing symptoms worse. When the trapped mucus is suctioned or relieved by irrigation or when I can finally clear it myself, my GERD and LPRD will usually resolve and my throat clearing will stop.

If you suffer from this symptom, don't feel as if you were either crazy or intentionally making others uncomfortable. While it is irritating to yourself and others around you, like any other symptom of sinus disease, it can be relieved through proper diagnosis and treatment.

Hoarseness

If enough mucus inflames the voice box, this area of the throat will swell, causing hoarseness and, in extreme cases, laryngitis. Worse, when the voice box becomes inflamed, polyps of the vocal cords can form. If you suffer from GERD and/or LPRD, the vocal cords can become irritated by acids from the stomach, which can itself cause hoarseness. GERD and LPRD can also cause swelling of the vocal cords and to the area behind the vocal cords, called the postglottic space. When your sinuses and GERD/LPRD are acting up, your vocal cords are getting hit from above (by the inflammatory postnasal drip) *and* from below (by the inflammatory acids coming up from the stomach).

Sore Throat

When mucus that is carrying infection, irritants, or allergens coats the throat, it can irritate its lining, which can make your throat red and sore and cause painful swallowing. Occasionally, pus will form on the membranes of the throat.

An infection of the sinuses can drain to Waldeyer's ring, the lymphatic tissue around the throat. This can cause tonsillitis and adenoiditis, especially in children. The adenoids typically disappear by the age of 5 years in a normal child. However, I've seen adults suffering from bad sinus disease whose adenoids are still present. I believe this is a result of the chronic infection.

Swollen Glands

In addition to Waldeyer's ring, the neck has about 300 tiny lymph nodes. These are imperceptible except when they become enlarged, either through infection or when a tumor appears. When this lymphatic tissue becomes enlarged, we refer to the condition as swollen glands. When this occurs, you may feel lumps or marble-like structures along the sides of your neck. The swollen glands can be subtle or may be so large that they can be viewed just by looking at the outside of the neck.

The tongue can also be affected. The tongue is a huge muscle that can swell during a severe allergic reaction or even a mild infection. In milder instances, you'll notice difficulty speaking. In severe instances, tongue swelling can cause you to stop breathing, and immediate medical attention is required. This swelling can lead to partial or total obstruction of the throat, although this is very rare.

Mouth Breathing

When your nose and sinuses become congested, the amount of air that can reach your lungs is compromised. The body's natural method to compensate for this lack of air intake is to allow us to breathe through our mouths. But mouth breathing is not normal: We are intended to breathe only through our nose. Yet many of us have been mouth breathers our whole lives.

Remember, the air that reaches our lungs must be heated, humidified, and filtered. The air that we breathe through our mouths will not have passed through the sinuses and, therefore, will not be cleansed before entering the lungs. Mouth breathers unknowingly allow dirt, infection, and inflammatory agents to enter their system, which is not good for the lungs or any part of the body.

You can tell when someone has trouble breathing through his or her nose because the mouth will be kept open, even slightly, at all times. This slight opening of the lips is referred to as breathing through "pursed" lips. Sometimes the obstruction is so bad that the mouth is always significantly open, giving the person an odd, quizzical look on his or her face. Chapped lips are another sign of a mouth breather. When you breathe through your mouth, the dry air will make your lips chapped. When your lips become chapped, you will have a tendency to lick them and this will make them more chapped. A mouth breather may have chapped lips even in the summer, when the air is moist with humidity.

Decreased or Absent Sense of Smell and/or Taste

When the olfactory nerve endings are inflamed the area around them is inflamed, the odors, scents, and smells from the outside world cannot be decoded. Your sense of smell will be dulled or may even disappear. Consequently, your sense of taste will suffer. Very often this dysfunction becomes gradually worse over time, and you may not even realize that you are having a problem with these two senses. However, it is not necessary to go through life without a clear sense of smell or taste. Like other symptoms, with proper treatment, these senses can usually be fully restored.

Dental and Facial Pain

The roots of the upper teeth often protrude into the maxillary sinus, where an infection can spread from the sinuses to the teeth, or vice versa. An infection that occurs in this manner can feel like pain in a single tooth or in a group of teeth. When this occurs, you may experience dental pain, which can vary from mild to severe. As well, an infection of the maxillary sinus can spread to the tooth root, which may require you to undergo a root canal.

The nerve that supplies sensation to the cheek is situated along the roof of the maxillary sinus. When this sinus is inflamed, you may experience pain when you press against your cheek or cheeks, if both cheek sinuses are involved. This infection can present itself as a headache, a sharp pain, or facial pressure. If the infection in the sinus is bad enough that it affects the maxillary nerve, it too can result in pain in one tooth or multiple upper teeth.

If you are experiencing any of these particular symptoms, be sure to discuss them with your primary-care physician or otolaryngologist, as well as your dentist.

Gingivitis, Halitosis (Bad Breath), and Dental Caries

When an infection in the sinuses spreads to the mouth, it may infect the gums and the teeth through your saliva. This infection can change the consistency of the saliva and you may develop bad breath, either all the time or just in the morning when your sinus infection is flaring. Dental decay can also occur, which may be mild but can become severe enough to rot your teeth.

Furthermore, the gums of mouth breathers are often dry, just like their chapped lips. This drying results from the dry air that you breathe through your mouth and a change in consistency that occurs in the saliva. Dry gums can bleed and turn red around the margins of the teeth. When this condition progresses, the gums can hurt when touched and/or when you eat. In fact, a dentist once told me that people who suffer from allergies have more dental problems than those who do not. I think that he had half the story correct: People that suffer from any blockage of the nose—including those who suffer from allergies, infection, inflammation, and/or anatomically narrowed sinus passageways—can suffer from dental problems at a higher frequency than the general population.

Sensation of a Bad/ Foul Smell: Parosmia

Some people can smell a bad or foul odor that travels with them throughout the day. Sometimes the smell is reminiscent of a moldy locker room. Occasionally it will be described as the smell of something burning. Often, the person notices the smell but can't figure out where it is coming from. While the person suffering from this symptom can actually be exuding this smelly odor, others around them may or may not pick up on the odor—and if they do, they may not mention it. For example, when my sinuses act up, my wife recognizes the odor first thing in the morning. She can differentiate the smell, not as "morning breath" but rather as the smell of infection.

This type of foul smell is almost always an indication of an infection. On rare occasions, it could also be an indication of a tumor near or on the olfactory nerve. Either way, if this is a constant symptom, you require medical attention and an immediate workup.

Nose Bleeds

If your sinuses and/or nose are infected, the inside of the nose will become dry as a result of the crusting and the change in air patterns stemming from the nasal obstruction. The infection can cause breaks in the membranes, and this can cause bleeding. You might see blood in your mucus. This bleeding can become more severe if the affected vessels are big enough or the damage to the membranes is significant. The medical term for a nose bleed is epistasis.

Nasal Polyps

Nasal polyps are benign growths or tumors that grow from the membranes of the sinuses or nose. It is theorized that polyps are caused by infection. It appears that under the polyp is infected bone. It is unclear whether the polyp stems from an original infection in the bone or the polyp infects the underlying bone. I believe that the infection starts in the membrane and spreads to the bone, causing a vicious cycle between the bone and the overlying tissue. The inflammation caused by the infection in the mucus and the bone causes the tissues of the nasal membranes to swell and welt. This swelling is called polypoid change. As the inflammation and swelling worsens, a polyp forms. When there are many polyps, the tissue looks like a bunch of grapes.

The only way to truly know that you have nasal polyps is from an examination of the membranes. However, most physicians are not able to tell the difference between polyps and swollen turbinates. It is best to go to an otolaryngologist, who will not only examine you directly but may order a computed tomography (CT) scan.

Papilloma

Papilloma are warts that form in the nose and/or the sinuses. There are two types of warts. The benign version is similar to those you may have on your hands or feet that grow outward. This papilloma is most commonly found on the septum or the turbinates. The second type is an inverted papilloma, which grows into the lining of the nose and sinuses. While inverted papilloma are usually benign as well, about 10 percent of them may transform into cancer.

All nasal and sinus warts are caused by the papilloma virus, which attacks the nasal and sinus membranes. Patients may note some bleeding because these growths often bleed. Papilloma usually occur on one side of the nose, and patients will often complain of one-sided obstruction. There is no medicine to treat this, and surgical removal is usually recommended. A CT scan can detect a mass consistent with papilloma, but ultimately the diagnosis must be made by biopsy and pathological examination.

Cancer

Cancer of the sinuses is rare but does occur. Usually the first sign is constant nasal obstruction or bleeding on one side of the nose. Some nasal cancers look like polyps, which is why it is important to be fully evaluated by an otolaryngologist. Cancer of the sinuses can be deadly if not diagnosed and treated early.

Ear Pain and Pressure

Very often an ear infection is caused by a sinus infection. The ears are connected to the back of the nose by the eustachian tubes that run along the outside walls of the nasopharynx. The eustachian tubes keep the pressure between the ears and the nose equal and maintain the pressure in the ear the same as that in the outside world, which is constantly changing. At birth, the eustachian tubes may be horizontal or even angle upward, but as we get older, the angle of the tubes changes so that the tube drains into the nasopharynx. If the nasopharynx becomes inflamed, the ears can feel clogged as the eustachian tubes become swollen. An infection with fluid buildup can occur in the middle ear, leading to hearing loss, ear pain, and pressure.

Hearing Loss, Tinnitus, and Vertigo

Hearing loss can be caused by many factors, including—as just noted—an infection or fluid buildup in the middle ear. This infection can also cause tinnitus, a constant ringing in the ear. A cholesteatoma, a benign tumor that develops from a pressure gradient, can form, causing the eardrum to suck in on itself. This destroys the eardrum, leading to hearing loss. The cholesteatoma can erode the bones in the middle ear, which also causes hearing loss. A cholesteatoma needs immediate surgical management. The middle ear is connected to the outside world through the eustachian tube. When an eustachian tube becomes swollen or blocked, the middle ear can no longer equalize pressure with the outside world. When this happens, you may experience the sensation of being under water (dull hearing), dizziness, vertigo, or a feeling of imbalance. The dizziness can range from feeling a little off balance to feeling as the room were spinning.

In addition, chronic ear pressure can lead to ear infections. For instance, bacteria from the sinuses can spread to the ear and result in an acute ear infection and muffled hearing. If the infection worsens, the ear can start to drain as it makes a hole in the eardrum. This discharge through the eardrum is usually a foul-smelling pus. When the infection is acute, you can experience severe pain. If the eardrum is stretched severely or too quickly, you may also experience ear pain from acute bleeding into the eardrum.

Sometimes the eustachian tube becomes enlarged. This can occur after significant weight loss or after an upper respiratory tract infection. When this occurs, air will pass too easily from the back of the nose to the middle ear, and you might experience the sensation of stuffiness in the head, and the chance of an infection spreading from the sinuses to the middle ear increases. You might also hear an internal grinding noise when you chew. Although this is an annoying symptom, it is usually not permanent. You may even start to hear yourself when you speak. This symptom is called echolalia, and usually resolves on its own.

Eye Problems

Many of us have experienced irritated, itchy, watery eyes during the allergy season. These very noticeable symptoms occur as a primary result of the allergic response. In addition, patients with allergies often have allergic shiners (especially noticeable in children) which are dark circles under the eyes. These shiners can also be caused by infection.

Aside from an allergic response, infection in the sinuses can cause myriad other eye complications, including facial swelling, eye protrusions, or an intraorbital (in the space of the eyeball) abscess. More drastically, tears forming in the tear glands in the upper eyelid flow down to the lower lid, drain into the inner aspect of your eye, and empty into the nasolacrimal duct into your nose. Inflammation of this tear duct (known as dacrocystitis) can lead to problems, including excessive tearing. When the infection backs up the duct into the corner of the eye, you may find yellow or green crust in the corners of your eyes. You might think that this is sleep dust, another "normal" part of life. However, it is a clear sign of an eye problem. Very often an ophthalmologist will diagnose dacryocystitis and keep dilating the duct without ever considering that the recurrent dacryocystitis may be caused by a sinus infection. This treatment will not produce results until the sinus infection has been properly treated.

If this infection goes farther into the eye, you can develop conjunctivitis, and your eyeball will appear red. Meibomitis is an inflammation of the meibomian glands (glands that form your tears). When this happens, you can see redness in the upper eyelids where the meibomian glands lie. The infection can lead to a sty, a small pimple forming in your eyelid. When the infection backs up the nasolacrimal duct, a film can cover the eye, causing the sensation of temporarily blurry vision.

Because of the position of the sphenoid sinuses, inflammation in this area can cause pain in the eye and in the top and back of the head. If the infection spreads to the area behind the eye, including the fat pad and the muscles that move your eye you may experience blurry vision, a limitation of eye movement, pain in your eye during movement, or a protrusion of your eye (called proptosis). The optic nerve, responsible for vision, and the oculomotor and trochlear nerves, responsible for controlling eye movement, also lie close to these sinuses; and an infection in the sphenoid sinuses can lead to double vision, reduced eye movement, and loss of vision—although this is very rare.

In some instances, an infection beginning in the sinuses can affect your overall vision. For example, I once had a patient named Mary, who was a 38-year-old accountant when she came to see me. She had chronic sinus infections, and her symptoms included yellow-green discharge, nasal obstruction, postnasal drip, swollen glands, decreased sense of smell, and sinus headaches. She had been on various medicines, including antibiotics, steroid nasal sprays, and antihistamines, yet her sinus problem was just getting worse.

After a careful examination, I knew that Mary required endoscopic sinus surgery to alleviate her symptoms. Immediately after surgery, Mary noticed a major change in her vision. Along with an immediate improvement in her breathing, her blurry vision disappeared. Mary explained that before the surgery she always had problems with her vision and often couldn't focus her eyes easily. Mary had always felt that there was a gauze film covering her eyes. She had never mentioned any eye problem to me before the surgery because she didn't think it was related. Yet after the surgery, her vision was completely clear.

SINUS SYMPTOMS THAT AFFECT THE LUNGS: ASTHMA AND BRONCHITIS

Remember that the nose and lungs are intimately connected, so an infection or inflammation that occurs in the nose can travel to the lungs, causing a host of significant conditions. Infected mucus can enter the lower airways through the trachea and the bronchi, leading to tracheitis and/or bronchitis. These conditions will manifest themselves in a range of symptoms, from a dry, heaving cough to difficulty breathing with a tightness of the chest.

When the smaller airways of the lung (alveoli) become involved, you may experience asthma symptoms. These symptoms range from mild wheezing to severe tightness or constriction of the chest, with severe shortness of breath. This reaction occurs when the lung tightens up so much that air cannot enter the lungs, and breathing can potentially stop. This is called status asthmaticus. Without treatment, asthma can be fatal. However, with the proper medication, asthma is completely controllable. If you or someone you know is suffering from tightness in the chest or persistent wheezing or coughing, please seek medical help right away.

When the lung tissue itself becomes infected and full of mucus that cannot be cleared through coughing, you may have developed pneumonia. In this instance, the infection actually invades the deep tissues of the lungs. The symptoms of pneumonia range from a persistent, ineffective cough to severe shortness of breath, and must be treated with prescription medication, which will clear the infection. Without proper treatment, pneumonia can also be fatal.

SEEMINGLY UNRELATED SYMPTOMS OF CAID

Fatigue

Feeling tired or run down is a medical condition and is not normal. When you experience chronic fatigue, you may feel as if you were always dragging or that you never get enough sleep. In severe cases, a doctor might diagnose your condition as chronic fatigue syndrome.

It is interesting that the number one cause for chronic fatigue syndrome is sinus disease. The initial sinus infection passes into the bloodstream, which can cause a transient bacteremia (infection in the bloodstream) leading to fatigue, and you may experience the same run down feeling as when you get the flu. The symptoms can be so debilitating that you can feel as if you couldn't get out of bed.

Fever

Inflammation that begins in the sinuses can affect your body temperature in two disparate ways. As the body reacts to the inflammation, it often raises your temperature, resulting in low-grade fever for some and high-grade fever for others. Usually, a high fever will alert you to the fact that your body is not functioning properly, and you will take the necessary steps to bring your fever under control. However, some people with chronic sinusitis run low-grade fevers every day and never recognize the change in body temperature.

Without proper treatment, the inflammatory process can become systemic when the infection moves into the bloodstream. This inflammatory response raises your body temperature as part of the reaction to bacteria in the bloodstream, and you may find that you sweat all night as a result. Some women confuse this symptom as an early sign of menopause but find that with proper treatment, this condition will disappear along with the other CAID symptoms. True menopausal night sweats will not go away through this type of treatment.

Sleep Disorders and Sleep Apnea

If you have a nasal obstruction that is more permanent on one side of the nose (e.g., a septal deviation, a nasal polyp, or scar tissue), you might find that you invariably choose to sleep with this side of the face closest to your pillow. Your nose will naturally become more congested because you are lying down, which is why people often complain that they are more congested at night. This congestion can lead to snoring. While you might not notice that you snore, your spouse or partner certainly does.

Chronic sinusitis and nasal obstruction can lead to sleep apnea, a condition in which you might stop breathing for a few seconds while you are sleeping. When this occurs, the heart does not get the proper concentration of oxygen. As a result of the apnea, these patients no longer get the rapid eye movement (REM) sleep they need, thereby compounding their fatigue. As stated earlier, there is strong evidence that sleep apnea is often referred to as a silent killer and is one of the causes of heart disease and stroke.

Stress

Stress can certainly result from dealing with many of the symptoms caused by sinus disease, allergies, and asthma. For example, constant throat clearing is stressful for both sufferers and the people around them. Snoring, sleep apnea, and fatigue will worsen stress. Conversely, stress can cause problems with sleep patterns.

Stress has also been found to worsen sinus problems. When you are stressed, your immunity can be compromised, making you more sensitive to sinus problems. And as your stress levels increase, you produce more stomach acids and your reflux can get worse, creating a vicious cycle, making you feel worse and emotionally anxious. Stress can flare asthma. And asthma can be quite stressful.

Depression

Sinus problems can prevent you from sleeping well, which can lead to fatigue. Combined with an overall feeling of sickness, fatigue can actually lead to depression. Many major conditions attributed to depression—including heart disease, weight gain, nervous tics, failure to conceive, and poor sexual performance—may also be linked to infected or inflamed sinuses. For instance, when people have significant sinus problems they can become fatigued, which will cause them to refrain from physical activity, and they can gain weight. Or depression from living with your CAID symptoms can cause overeating, which can also lead to weight gain. This weight gain can cause further depression. It can also worsen sleep apnea, making you more tired and thus more depressed. If you are experiencing the signs and symptoms of clinical depression as well as the signs and symptoms of sinus disease and are currently taking medication or seeing a psychiatrist, please discuss your sinus problems with your doctors. Working together with an otolaryngologist, your medical team can better cure your depression.

Meningitis, Encephalitis, and Brain Abscess

Meningitis, encephalitis, and brain abscess are rare complications of sinus infection. However, they can be life threatening and need to be treated immediately. Each of these infections is caused by complications of sinus disease and begins with symptoms that include headaches, fever, stiff neck, behavioral changes, and loss of concentration. The carotid artery, which carries the blood supply to the brain, runs along the outside wall of the sphenoid sinus; and the veins that drain the brain of deoxygenated blood end in the cavernous sinus, which is located behind the sphenoid sinus. As a result of the close proximity of these important vascular structures to the sphenoid sinus and the fact that this sinus is under the brain, a sphenoid sinus infection can spread to the brain quite easily. The frontal sinus sits in front of the brain, and the roof of the ethmoid sinus is the floor of the brain; therefore, infection in these areas can also spread to the brain. Furthermore, the blood vessels that supply the nose are connected to the blood vessels that supply the brain, so an infection of the nose can spread to the brain. Although rare, a brain abscess can form from an infection in any of these areas or a thrombosis of the cavernous sinus can occur as a result of a sphenoid sinus infection.

The number one cause of meningitis is sinus infection. Infection of the nose and sinuses are especially dangerous to the brain because an infection can travel upstream through the veins in the nose, which, unlike most veins, do not have valves. Any microfracture in the bone separating the sinuses from the brain can allow infection to travel to the brain or the surrounding tissues, leading to meningitis. Any small tear in the brain's covering (the dura) can lead to encephalitis. Furthermore, if the infection travels through the venous drainage into the brain, a brain abscess can occur.

GERD and Other Digestive Conditions

The symptoms of GERD include heartburn, indigestion, reflux, and belching. If you experience these symptoms along with any of the sinus infection symptoms just described, it is important that you see a specialist who understands the link between these disease processes.

When GERD occurs, the stomach contents rise above the junction between the stomach and the esophagus. When they reach the voice box and drop into the lung, the condition is LPRD. The acids may even rise above the pharynx (throat) and actually reach the nose and sinuses. There are other inflammatory bowel disease processes that affect the GI tract, including Crohn's disease and ulcerative colitis. The symptoms of Crohn's disease, which are similar to those of ulcerative colitis, often include fatigability. There also may be a palpable mass in the colon with Crohn's disease.

For instance, my patient Monte suffered from sinus disease and headaches that kept him up at night. He also experienced bad gastroesophageal reflux. I told him that his GERD was brought on by his sinus infections. The mucus that pools in his sinuses eventually drips into his throat, is swallowed, and passes into his stomach. This causes his reflux to act up. He noted that when his postnasal drip worsened, his reflux got worse. Once he began to follow the prescribed regimen, his symptoms virtually disappeared. He is now getting enough sleep, no longer suffers from headaches, and does not experience acid reflux.

GERD/LPRD and asthma are known to be clinically related. Sometimes, asthma is the first symptom noted in a GERD/LPRD diagnosis. If GERD/LPRD is not properly or is incompletely treated, then reflux of stomach acid can enter the lung, setting off asthma symptoms. The acids from the stomach inflame the lining of the lungs, and you may start wheezing. These acids can also cause a chemical tracheitis or bronchitis, resulting in a chronic cough or throat clearing. Treating the GERD/LPRD appropriately at the onset may prevent the asthma and at the very least will improve the likelihood that the reflux will not cause significant inflammation to the trachea, bronchi, or lung.

SINUS SYMPTOMS AND CHILDREN

I believe that children develop CAID symptoms just the same as adults, but they often go undetected by pediatricians, who are not adequately trained in this condition. Most parents typically ignore a runny stuffy nose, swollen glands, cough, or hoarse voice until a significant fever is produced. I have met parents who talk about these symptoms as if they were normal or an expected part of childhood. But once again, these conditions are not normal. Untreated chronic sinus problems are not just uncomfortable for your young children but can cause life-long damage.

The Next Step to Healing

Now that you recognize and understand your symptoms, you should realize that you are not alone. Many people suffer from CAID, most of whom never seek proper medical treatment. Others will treat some symptoms and not others. But it is only when the entire disease process is treated effectively that you will get the best possible result. Comprehensive medical care can often allow all of your symptoms to disappear as you maintain control over your health.

While it is true that sinus disease is usually benign, it can ruin your quality of life. Some people believe that they may have a constant cold or an allergy, when in fact their condition is much worse. These patients live with chronic headaches or fatigue, thinking that they must forever endure these symptoms. Some patients feel that it is normal not to have developed a sense of smell or taste or, worse, may not even realize that these senses are diminished. All of these people are facing potentially significant health problems. Until these symptoms are diagnosed properly and then treated, you will never be aware of how much better, fuller, and richer your life can be.

The rest of this book addresses the specific branches of CAID and how each of their symptoms and conditions are related to specific aspects of this greater disease process. The next step to reclaiming your good health is to understand how these diseases affect your body and what you need to do to treat them effectively.

CHAPTER 3

DIAGNOSING YOUR SYMPTOMS: THE CAID TEST

Now that you understand the signs and symptoms that may occur from any of the limbs of chronic airway-digestive inflammatory disease (CAID), the next step is to accurately pinpoint which of the limbs you are currently experiencing, and where the cascade of symptoms began. For example, you may know that you suffer from seasonal allergies. Every fall, you might experience dry, itchy eyes, nasal congestion, and a constant feeling of postnasal drip. None of these symptoms really holds you back from your daily life, and knowing that they are "just" the result of allergies, you leave them alone, hoping that they will disappear once the leaves are finally swept away in late November.

Yet one October day you wake up with a pounding headache, and you are so fatigued that you can't get out of bed. Your temperature is well above normal, your reflux is acting up, and you are feeling miserable. What happened? While your initial reaction might be to connect these more severe symptoms to a cold or the beginnings of the flu, in reality your untreated allergy symptoms spawned an infection in your sinuses. Had you treated your allergy symptoms earlier, you may have forgone these later, more distressing symptoms of CAID. It is scenarios like this one that make having a proper diagnosis—and following up with the necessary treatment—paramount.

What Causes CAID?

When a doctor makes a diagnosis, he or she has in mind a list of potential ailments that may be appropriate to your symptoms. This list is called a differential diagnosis. From the differential diagnosis, the doctor can determine which treatments will best resolve your symptoms. For you to develop your own differential diagnosis, you have to think like a physician.

Following is the differential diagnosis tree for the nasal and sinus problems associated with CAID. Each of the main causes is broken into subsections, based on the likely underlying cause of the problem. For example, we know that nasal and sinus problems can be caused by an infection, an irritation, an allergy, or an anatomical defect. If we suspect an infection, we then need to identify it by its origin: bacterium, fungus (mold), and/or virus.

DIFFERENTIAL DIAGNOSIS

Infectious
- Bacterial
- Fungal
- Viral

Irritants
- Car exhaust
- Chemicals
- Cigarette smoke
- Cleaning products
- Industry-related products
- New carpeting
- Paints
- Perfume
- Stress
- Foods

Allergic
- Environmental
- Foods

Traumatic/Anatomic Variants
- Nasal and/or sinus structures
- Septum
- Iatrogenic (previous surgery)

DETERMINING YOUR DIAGNOSIS

For you to obtain the right treatment, you need to determine which of these underlying causes is aggravating your system and causing your CAID symptoms. As you can see from the differential diagnosis tree, there are so many underlying causes of CAID that making the right diagnosis for each sufferer can be very difficult.

When you seek medical treatment, the first thing a doctor will ask is how you are feeling. What the doctor is really asking is for you to list your symptoms so he or she can narrow down the choices from a differential diagnosis tree. Your physician will then do a complete physical examination, including proper testing if necessary. All of these pieces then fit together to determine an accurate diagnosis.

THE PATIENT DETECTIVE

Your role in accurately conveying your symptoms is probably the most important aspect of the diagnosis. I tell my patients all the time that they are the best resource in finding a solution for their problems. I count on my patient's detective skills: Without them, I could potentially be making a faulty diagnosis.

For instance, the term *headache* denotes a symptom that is related to many different diagnoses. Headaches can be diagnosed as vascular, migraine, infectious, traumatic, tension, or sinus, among others, depending on their pattern and associated complaints, such as location, duration, and severity. To make things more confusing, each of these types of headaches can sometimes have overlapping patterns. Worse, you may be suffering from more than one type of headache.

For the physician to make the most accurate diagnosis, you must accurately communicate the subtle nuances of exactly what and how you are feeling. At the same time, your doctor must carefully listen to your description. For example, many people suffer from sinus headaches, yet incorrectly label this symptom as a migraine. They may have learned that a migraine occurs when there is pain located behind the eyes and in the forehead, and this pain causes distorted vision, light sensitivity, and a headache that radiates to one side of the head. Yet these same symptoms can also be attributed to a sinus headache or a sinus headache that precedes a migraine headache. If your physician takes your self-diagnosis of migraine headaches without probing you to describe your symptoms, you may be incorrectly treated for the wrong type of headache for years to follow. When this treatment doesn't work, you won't realize that it was your incorrect reporting or your physician's misdiagnosis that actually caused the misunderstanding.

Unfortunately, people suffering from CAID are routinely misdiagnosed. In fact, CAID is one of the most misdiagnosed medical problems. Often it is overlooked as a cause of chronic fatigue syndrome, headaches, and/or snoring. For instance, my patient Jaclyn is a 28-year-old lawyer who spent an entire year searching for treatment for what she thought was a constant cold. When she finally came into my office, she told me that she suffered from painful headaches that seemed to move around her face: Often they occurred in her forehead, yet at other times she felt the pain in her cheeks and around her eyes. Jaclyn was hoarse and experienced swollen glands, ear congestion, and constant fatigue. She also suffered from intermittent neck stiffness. She regularly missed work owing to her symptoms and never found any relief with over-the-counter medications.

Jaclyn was so uncomfortable that she went to a variety of doctors, including an internist, an allergist, and even an ear, nose, and throat (ENT) specialist; no one was able to help her. Her allergist performed routine testing and told her that she did not have allergies, yet he prescribed antihistamines. When none of the traditional medications worked, Jaclyn began experimenting with alternative medicine. She went to an acupuncturist who treated her with cupping to the point that her back looked as if she had been beaten.

After Jaclyn finished her story, we discussed the details of her symptoms and the treatments she had already received. I followed up our conversation with a comprehensive workup, including a complete family history and a thorough physical examination. I sent her for a computed tomography (CT) scan and performed an endoscopic examination. The results from my physical examination and from the medical history pointed toward a diagnosis of CAID, manifesting in a problem with her sinuses. My findings were compatible with the initial allergist: The underlying cause was not related to allergies (which was why the prescribed antihistamines never provided her relief). Yet I saw that Jaclyn's sinus passageways were structurally too narrow, an anatomical condition she had her entire life but that never bothered her until her nasal membranes became inflamed from what I could only guess was a long-term infection. I recommended that, while surgery would be an effective solution, we should first try a new regimen of prescription medications and chiropractic treatment. Luckily for Jaclyn, she was able to find relief by following this protocol.

Today Jaclyn is able to breathe freely and no longer has sinus headaches or neck pain. She subsequently had a baby and told me that she was enjoying motherhood, free of the suffering caused by her sinus problems.

The CAID Quiz

While the CAID conditions of sinus disease, pulmonary disease (asthma), gastroesophageal reflux disease (GERD), and laryngopharyngeal reflux disease (LPRD) are all linked, it is equally important to differentiate among each to administer optimum treatment. The following self-guided quiz will facilitate the process so that you can organize your symptoms and see which treatments are necessary. Depending on your answers, you will be able to conclusively tell whether you are suffering from sinus disease, allergies, asthma, or GERD, or any combination. You will also be able to discern which of these processes triggers your symptoms, so that with your physician you will be able to treat the underlying problem before more serious symptoms occur.

The first set of questions cover general issues associated with CAID.

They are the most common symptoms of the disease. Rate each of the following symptoms on a scale from 0 to 5: 0 means the symptom does not exist, 1 means a minimal presence, 2 means often bothersome, 3 means affecting you daily, 4 means affecting your lifestyle, and 5 means debilitating. Circle the appropriate number after each question.

PART ONE

Sinus Disease

1. I feel tired and run down. 0 1 2 3 4 5
2. I experience facial swelling and puffiness. 0 1 2 3 4 5
3. I have dark circles under or around my eyes. 0 1 2 3 4 5
4. I feel that I've lost my sense of smell or taste. 0 1 2 3 4 5
5. I find myself sniffling. 0 1 2 3 4 5
6. I have a funny feeling in my ears. 0 1 2 3 4 5
7. I have bad breath. 0 1 2 3 4 5
8. I have dental problems: cavities, root canal,
   and/or periodontal work. 0 1 2 3 4 5
9. I have experienced hearing loss. 0 1 2 3 4 5
10. I have experienced sleep apnea. 0 1 2 3 4 5
11. I have facial pain. 0 1 2 3 4 5
12. I have frequent headaches. 0 1 2 3 4 5
13. I have trouble breathing through my nose. 0 1 2 3 4 5
14. I have had eye swelling even to the point
    of closure. 0 1 2 3 4 5
15. I frequently cough. 0 1 2 3 4 5
16. I experience blocked tear ducts. 0 1 2 3 4 5
17. I experience dizziness. 0 1 2 3 4 5
18. I experience dry eyes. 0 1 2 3 4 5
19. I experience excessive tearing. 0 1 2 3 4 5
20. I experience nasal congestion. 0 1 2 3 4 5
21. I experience postnasal drip. 0 1 2 3 4 5
22. I experience sinus pressure. 0 1 2 3 4 5
23. I have been diagnosed with tinnitus (ringing
    or buzzing in ears). 0 1 2 3 4 5

24. I find crust in the corners of my eyes. 0 1 2 3 4 5
25. I have a runny nose. .0 1 2 3 4 5
26. I have a sore throat. 0 1 2 3 4 5
27. I have swollen glands. 0 1 2 3 4 5
28. I have watery eyes. .0 1 2 3 4 5
29. I have chapped lips year-round. 0 1 2 3 4 5
30. I'm constantly clearing my throat. 0 1 2 3 4 5
31. I'm frequently hoarse. 0 1 2 3 4 5
32. I've been diagnosed with conjunctivitis
    (pink eye). 0 1 2 3 4 5
33. I've been told that I snore. 0 1 2 3 4 5
34. My ears are clogged. 0 1 2 3 4 5
35. My nostrils are crusty. 0 1 2 3 4 5

Results for Sinus Disease

If your score is less than 5 points, you are probably not suffering from any aspect of CAID. You might be experiencing a cold or, at worst, the flu. If your score was more than 5, read Chapter 4 on sinus disease. But first, continue with the remainder of the test to determine the underlying cause of your CAID.

The following sections will help you determine your personal diagnosis: Is the cause infectious, an irritant, anatomical, allergic, or a combination of these? Depending on the results of the tests, you will be able to determine which limb of CAID is causing your symptoms. Rank each of the following symptoms on a scale of 0 to 5: 0 means the symptom does not exist, 1 means a minimal presence, 2 means often bothersome, 3 means affecting you daily, 4 means affecting your lifestyle, and 5 means debilitating.

PART TWO: DISTINGUISHING CAID SYMPTOMS

Allergy

1. I frequently sneeze. .0 1 2 3 4 5
2. I experience nasal stuffiness. 0 1 2 3 4 5
3. I experience sinus pressure. 0 1 2 3 4 5

4. I have hives or a rash. 0 1 2 3 4 5
5. I have itchy eyes. 0 1 2 3 4 5
6. I have experienced asthma more than
   once in my life. 0 1 2 3 4 5
7. My skin is itchy without being dry. 0 1 2 3 4 5
8. My symptoms come and go with the changing
   of the seasons. 0 1 2 3 4 5
9. The area around my eyes and nose seems swollen. .0 1 2 3 4 5
10. I have dark circles under or around my eyes. 0 1 2 3 4 5
11. I feel run down. 0 1 2 3 4 5

Results for Allergy

If your score is less than 5 points, you are probably not suffering from allergies, and your CAID is stemming from another cause. If your score was more than 5, read chapter 4, which covers sinus disease, and Chapter 5, which discusses allergies. Continue with the remainder of the test to make certain that you are not also affected by another limb of CAID.

Asthma

1. I have felt myself wheezing. 0 1 2 3 4 5
2. I have heard myself wheezing without the aid
   of a stethoscope. 0 1 2 3 4 5
3. I frequently feel tightness in my chest. 0 1 2 3 4 5
4. I often experience shortness of breath. 0 1 2 3 4 5
5. I often feel short of breath or wheeze during
   or after exercise. 0 1 2 3 4 5
6. I often cough for periods at a time. 0 1 2 3 4 5

Results for Asthma

Asthma symptoms should not be taken lightly. If your score is less than 3 points, you are probably not suffering from asthma, and your CAID is stemming from another cause. If your score was more than 5, read Chapter 4, which covers sinus disease, and Chapter 6, which discusses asthma. Continue with the remainder of the test to make certain that you are not also affected by another limb of CAID. Asthma and GERD are intimately linked, so if your score in this section is high, it is especially important to finish the remainder of the quiz.

GERD

1. I belch often. 0 1 2 3 4 5
2. I cough at night when I lay down. 0 1 2 3 4 5
3. I have a sour taste in my mouth. 0 1 2 3 4 5
4. I have bad breath. 0 1 2 3 4 5
5. I experience heart burn. 0 1 2 3 4 5
6. I experience hoarseness. 0 1 2 3 4 5
7. I experience indigestion. 0 1 2 3 4 5
8. I experience reflux. 0 1 2 3 4 5
9. I have a sore throat. 0 1 2 3 4 5
10. I'm often clearing my throat. 0 1 2 3 4 5

Results for GERD

If your score is less than 5 points, you are probably not suffering from GERD, and your CAID is stemming from another cause. If your score was more than 5, read Chapter 4, which covers sinus disease, and Chapter 7, which discusses GERD.

Genetic Predisposition

I strongly believe that anyone who suffers from any limb of CAID is experiencing symptoms because of a genetic predisposition. In other words, CAID sufferers are easily affected by their underlying problem primarily because they are genetically programmed to have a specific reaction to that particular irritant. For example, if the symptom quiz suggested that you may have experienced an allergic reaction, either this allergy runs in your family or you are genetically susceptible to it. This includes all reactions, whether the irritant is allergic, infectious, immunological, or primarily inflammatory in nature. One day genetic research will uncover the answer to the genetic defects that cause us to suffer from the symptoms of CAID. Until then, it is helpful to understand that genetics may explain why some people are affected and others are not.

The Next Step

Based on the results from the quiz, read the chapters that correspond to your specific symptoms. Discuss these symptoms with your doctor, who will determine if you need to see a specialist. Once under a doctor's care, retake this quiz every 3 months to see if there is improvement. Note if new symptoms occur and if symptoms are lessened. Record your scores and compare them over time to see if the treatment is working.

MEETING WITH A PHYSICIAN

As you can see, CAID is complex, and its diagnosis is multifaceted. That is why it is important for anyone who suffers from one or more limbs of CAID to be managed by a team of physicians. I believe that an ENT specialist (otolaryngologist) should be considered the leader of the specialist team. Most internists will admit that they have only the minimum of schooling in sinus issues, but the majority of their patients have these problems. Conversely, ENTs have the most schooling in these issues. It is important for your ENT to keep your primary-care physician updated as to the treatment that is being prescribed.

If you now identify that you are suffering from severe sinus pain, you should seek treatment from an otolaryngologist who can treat your condition with medical and/or surgical remedies. If you have been seen by an ENT before and you have not received satisfactory treatment, you may want to seek out another ENT who specializes in sinus problems. Your primary-care physician, or even a general ENT, can refer you to someone who he or she considers an expert in this field.

Once you make an appointment with an ENT, it will be helpful for you to obtain all applicable information from your current physician(s) describing your past history, any testing, and all treatments provided—both medical (bring in a list of all of the medicines that you have taken) and surgical (bring in all the operative reports). You should also bring any imaging studies (X-rays, CT scans) that you may have had. It is much more helpful to bring in the original films along with any written reports, as the report will not usually give your ENT as much information as the films themselves. If you have had previous surgery, the surgical reports are also helpful.

Your initial visit to an otolaryngologist should be relatively uniform. In my office, every examination begins with patient questionnaires, a thorough medical history, and a physical examination. While I'm focusing on patients' ears, noses, throats, and chests, I'm also evaluating their overall appearance. I note if they are well kept, evaluate whether they are overweight, and determine if they breathe with an open or closed mouth. I evaluate their skin color and the general health of their skin. I listen to the quality of their voice, noting if they are hyponasal or hoarse. I explore their facial features and check for swelling around the eyes and puffiness around the face, over the forehead, and in the cheeks. I look for black-and-blue marks around the eyes. I perform an evaluation of the eyes and tap or press on the sinus areas for tenderness. I look at the lids for swelling or redness, the whites of the eyes for discoloration or redness, and the corners of the eyes for crusting. I look for tearing, note the position of the eyeballs, and the way that their eyes move. I look at the nose for swelling, creases, crusting, or bleeding and then look into the nose for discolored mucus, blood, crusting, scabbing, and dryness. I note the color of the membranes and the shape of the nasal valve and the septum and see if the turbinates are swollen or obstructive. I also determine if there are any polyps or papilloma.

Next I look at the mouth and throat. I look for a change in the thickness and color of the membranes and look for postnasal drip. I examine the membranes throughout and smell the breath. I look at the teeth and gums to see if there is dryness and/or bleeding or redness. I look at the size of the tonsils and note the way the palate lines up with the back of the throat. I look at the uvula (which hangs down in the back of the throat). I feel the neck for swollen glands, thyroid enlargement, or any enlarged lumps. If patients complain of pain in their teeth, I may tap the teeth to identify an inflamed tooth root.

I examine the ears for wax, note the shape of the ear canal, and look at the quality of the eardrum. Last, I listen to their lungs to detect noisy breathing or wheezing.

Of course, it may be important to evaluate the nose and the sinuses more thoroughly. I usually do this after a course of medical therapy has been tried. As well, I try to have a recent CT scan available at the time that I perform an endoscopic exam so that I may compare the films to my findings. However, your ENT may perform the examination and tests in a different manner. For an endoscopic evaluation, I use the most advanced diagnostic tools that are currently available, including an endoscope, which is a special fiber-optic instrument used to examine the interior of the nose and sinuses. I find that an endoscopic examination provides the most reliable visualization of many of the accessible areas of the sinus drainage pathways and can quickly allow one to determine if any of these areas are blocked.

To do this procedure, I first numb the nasal cavity with a combination of a decongestant and a topical anesthetic spray. For evaluation of the nose, I prefer to use a rigid nasal endoscope, and I gently place it in each nostril one at a time. During this examination, I can see if there is infection, polyp formation, and/or structural abnormalities that may cause obstruction in both the nose and the sinuses. In patients who have had previous sinus surgery, I can often see directly into the sinuses and evaluate scarring, infection, polyp formation, and closure of the passageways. Evaluation of the nasopharynx and the eustachian tubes gives us additional information. During the endoscopic examination you may feel a firm pressure in the nose, which is slightly uncomfortable, but this is usually not painful.

For patients who complain of hoarseness and/or symptoms consistent with LPRD/GERD, I prefer to use a flexible fiber-optic nasopharyngolaryngoscope to evaluate the voice box. Although on occasion I have used a rigid laryngoscope.

If I recognize that an infection exists, and the patient has recently finished a course of antibiotics, I may take a culture sample under endoscopic visualization and send it to a laboratory for further investigation. A laboratory may be able to identify a fungus or a resistant organism (a bacterium that is not sensitive to antibiotic treatment). For the culture, I swab the affected area to obtain a small sample of infected mucus. This sample is then placed in a tube containing culture medium. Many physicians run the swab directly across a glass plate (called "plating a culture") where the bacteria or fungi will grow. The swab that I send to the lab will be plated there. If bacteria are present, the bacteria will start growing on the plate. Once the organism is identified, the lab can treat the bacteria with various antibiotics to determine which one will yield the best results. If the bacteria continue to grow when placed near a particular antibiotic, then the organism is resistant to that specific antibiotic. Fungal cultures can be performed as well. Tests for major basic protein (MBP) can also be taken by sending your mucus to a lab. MBP is present as a result of fungal sinusitis.

Unfortunately, cultures are not always as accurate as we would like them to be. At times, they yield a false-positive result (cultures that are positive because of contamination although they should really be negative), or a false-negative result (which means that the culture is negative even though bacteria or fungus is really present). For example, a false negative may be found if the patient is on a course of antibiotics.

There are many physicians who feel that cultures are a waste of time. I believe that cultures have their place. For example, if a patient is feeling better but a culture shows a resistant organism, then perhaps a continuation of antibiotic treatment is warranted. In the end, I always put more weight on the clinical picture than on the culture.

If I notice significant nasal obstruction and/or have been told by the patient of repeated infections that have not cleared with medicine or if I suspect a tumor or polyps or cancer, then I will order a CT scan. A CT scan is a very good way to evaluate the sinuses. Patients may obtain a CT scan at a radiology imaging center, a hospital (these scanners are made by various companies including GE, Hitachi, Philips, Siemens, and Toshiba), and in some cases at their physician's offices using a smaller version called the MiniCAT (made by Xoran Technology). Each type of scanner has benefits and limitations. Today's CT scan units are not as confining as they used to be and are more comfortable for the patient. The larger scanners operate with the patient lying on a table and have more capabilities than the smaller versions. Of course CT scan testing, like all testing, is not perfect, although the technology has improved greatly over the years. CT scans show the shadow of the disease but cannot pinpoint the exact nature of the disease. In fact, they occasionally don't spot the disease altogether, and the scan may appear normal. For this reason, the diagnosis of sinus disease should be based on a comprehensive history and a thorough physical examination including an endoscopic examination, as well as the CT scan.

If during the medical history I am told of a diminished sense of smell or taste, I might want to order a magnetic resonance imaging (MRI) study because this is the best way to evaluate the brain and the olfactory nerve. An MRI scan can be obtained at a radiology facility or at a hospital. These scanners are made by various companies including GE, Hitachi, Philips, Siemens, and Toshiba. If the history suggests an immunological, infectious, or inflammatory cause, various blood tests should be ordered. These blood tests might include the following:

- Complete blood count (CBC) with a differential, which means we look at the level and activity of the types of white blood cells
- Erythrocyte sedimentation rate (ESR), which measures an inflammatory response
- Immunoglobulin G (IgG) and its subclasses and IgE, which are the immunoglobulins affiliated with infection and allergy
- Immunoglobulins A and M, which are affiliated with fighting infection
- Antinuclear antibody (ANA) and antineutrophil cytoplasmic antibody (ANCA), both of which measure antibodies in the blood
- Lyme titer, if there has been exposure to deer ticks
- Angiotensin-converting enzyme (ACE) level, which is highly suggestive of sarcoid disease

When I get the results from the various tests, I often consult with other specialists to meet each patient's individual needs. In my practice, I manage the care of my patients, referring them to a variety of medical specialists, including allergist/immunologists, pulmonologists, infectious disease specialists, endocrinologists, ophthalmologists, and rheumatologists. Should the patient suffer from allergies, I work with an allergist (either medically or otolaryngologically trained) who practices allergy/immunology. Either training for allergy specialization is fine. I recommend to the allergist that he or she do a complete allergy workup and, if needed, recommend that he or she perform immunology testing. If the patient suffers from asthma, I like to work with either a pulmonologist or an allergist/immunologist who specializes in asthma, both types of specialists can perform a pulmonary function test. This test analyzes the patient's lung capacity.

If I have a suspicion that the infectious agent(s) may be more complex, I might ask for some advice from an infectious disease specialist. If there are underlying eye problems, I will consult an ophthalmologist (eye doctor). If the patient is complaining of different types of headaches I will send him or her to a neurologist. When there is a question about rheumatological disease involvement as in the case of lupus, sarcoid or wegener's granulomatosis disease, then I ask a rheumatologist to consult. If there are concerns regarding a patient's metabolism, I will refer him or her to an endocrinologist.

If a patient is complaining of sinus headaches along with neck and back pain, I will send him or her to a chiropractor or acupuncturist. I will consult with a dentist if there is an infection present in the gums or upper teeth. Last, if diet seems to be an issue, either a traditional or holistic nutritionist will be able to address the problem and offer individual solutions for food plans.

Moreover, I advise patients to make sure either they or the otolaryngologist keeps their primary-care physician—usually an internist, family practitioner, pediatrician, or osteopath—in the loop to manage their total care. The primary-care physician is ultimately the one doctor responsible for your overall health, so he or she needs to be kept abreast of diagnoses and treatments being administered by any specialists.

AFTER AN ENDOSCOPIC EXAM

Refrain from drinking or eating for at least ½ hour after the examination because your throat will still be numb. Do not drink or eat any hot foods for approximately 2 hours after the examination because you may have decreased temperature sensitivity during this period. After 1 hour, the numbness should be mostly resolved. The examination may cause minimal bleeding and may result in a minor headache, which usually resolves by the next day. However, this is rare.

PART TWO

THE FIVE LIMBS
OF CAID

CHAPTER 4

TREATING SINUS DISEASE FOR OPTIMUM HEALTH

Sinusitis is the first limb of chronic airway-digestive inflammatory disease (CAID), and like CAID, can be caused by infection (bacterial, fungal/mold, or viral), allergies, environmental elements (car exhaust, cigarette smoke, or mold) and/or the anatomical narrowing of the sinuses. The diagnosis of sinusitis refers to an inflammation of the sinus membranes, whereas rhinitis means inflammation of the lining of the nose and turbinates. Inflammation can occur in either of these areas alone or simultaneously: Your doctor might have used the term *rhinosinusitis* to describe your condition.

The signs and symptoms of sinusitis or rhinosinusitis can vary for each sufferer. It's not uncommon for someone to misdiagnose his or her symptoms as a cold or the flu and self-medicate improperly. Therefore, it's always important to check with a doctor before taking any over-the-counter (OTC) remedies. Although you may be treating your symptoms with these medicines, you'll never get rid of the underlying cause and you will continue to feel sick. Your doctor is better equipped to accurately diagnose your problem and then to prescribe the proper remedy so that you will get back on your feet faster.

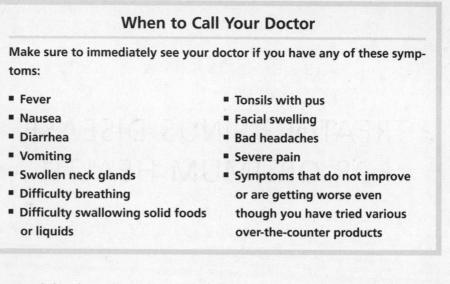

When to Call Your Doctor

Make sure to immediately see your doctor if you have any of these symptoms:

- Fever
- Nausea
- Diarrhea
- Vomiting
- Swollen neck glands
- Difficulty breathing
- Difficulty swallowing solid foods or liquids

- Tonsils with pus
- Facial swelling
- Bad headaches
- Severe pain
- Symptoms that do not improve or are getting worse even though you have tried various over-the-counter products

Luckily, there have been amazing advances in the diagnosis and treatment of all of the limbs of CAID, including sinusitis. There are many new medicines and combinations of medical treatments that can offer you long-lasting relief.

Understanding Your Diagnosis

There are three general types of sinusitis or rhinosinusitis: acute, acute recurrent, and chronic. While all three types of sinusitis or rhinosinusitis are caused by inflammation, the duration of the inflammation defines your problem. See which of the following descriptions best describes your current state of health.

ACUTE SINUSITIS

Acute sinusitis is defined as a short-term condition, lasting no more than 2 weeks, whether or not it has been treated. The signs and symptoms of acute sinusitis include facial pain/pressure, nasal obstruction, nasal discharge, diminished sense of smell, and cough. In addition, you may experience fever, chills, bad breath, fatigue, dental pain, swollen or tender neck glands, and sore throat. When an acute viral infection is present the nasal discharge is usually clear. A bacterial infection can occur on top of the viral infection and is often accompanied by a yellow, green, or tan/brown nasal discharge.

This initial hit of inflammation would probably lead you to believe that you had come down with a simple cold. You may have been right if your symptoms were relieved within 24–72 hours, whether or not you treated them. But colds should not last more than 2 weeks: if your symptoms persist, you probably have acute sinusitis.

There are more than 200 different viruses that are known to cause the symptoms of the common cold. Rhinoviruses affect the inside the nose and cause an estimated 30–35 percent of all adult colds. These types of viruses seldom produce serious illness.

Treating Acute Sinusitis and Rhinosinusitis

Unfortunately, there are no medicines today that fight viral sinus infections. The decongestants, cough suppressants, and fever/pain medications will only make you feel more comfortable through the healing phase. Antibiotics are never administered to treat either the common cold or viral acute sinusitis. Unfortunately, many patients expect their physician to prescribe an antibiotic whenever they feel sick. However, this line of thinking is not only wrong but potentially dangerous. First, antibiotics are not able to clear a viral infection. Second, unwarranted exposure to antibiotics can lead to resistance, so that they won't work when you really need them. If your physician tells you that your sinuses have flared because of a viral infection, then you should be happy that he or she is not giving you an antibiotic unnecessarily.

However, it is possible that the day after you see your doctor you may develop a change in the color of your nasal discharge from clear to yellow or green, which would indicate a bacterial superinfection. This occurs when there is a bacterial infection on top of a viral infection. It does not mean that your cold "turned into" a bacterial infection. An acute bacterial infection might be present if your symptoms last for more than 24–72 hours or worsen over 5–7 days. If this is the case, your doctor will then need to see you again and prescribe an antibiotic. Usually, a course of 7–14 days of antibiotics will clear up any acute bacterial infection.

Acute sinusitis responds well to the same treatment regimen that you would follow if you had a cold. If your physician feels that you have a viral infection, it is best to do the following:

- Drink plenty of fluids to keep mucus thin and flowing.
- Get plenty of rest, as much as 12 hours or more a night.
- Take OTC oral decongestants to get relief.

OTC decongestants, such as pseudoephedrine, work well on a short-term basis over a few days. I caution you not to take them long term because they have stimulant-like properties and have potentially serious side effects on the heart and prostate. If you have diabetes, heart disease, high blood pressure, and/or prostate or thyroid problems or are taking any medicines like monoamine oxidase (MAO) inhibitors (drugs taken for depression, psychiatric or emotional conditions, or Parkinson's disease) consult your doctor before taking a decongestant because it can lead to serious complications.

- Seek medical attention after 24 hours if a nasal decongestant spray does not provide significant improvement.

Topical (spray) decongestants provide temporary relief for a stuffy nose but should not be used for more than 24 hours, after which the body will fight back by rebounding. This means your nose will swell and produce even more thick mucus. If you continue to use a nasal decongestant, your condition will slowly worsen and your nose will likely become more congested than it was originally. Nasal decongestant sprays can also damage the blood supply to the nose and sinuses and interfere with cilia function after repetitive use. I do not recommend use of a topical decongestant for more than 24 hours unless under a physician's care. These can be very dangerous products if used incorrectly.

- Take an OTC anti-inflammatory, antipyretic, or analgesic agent (such as aspirin, ibuprofen or acetaminophen) for relief from fever and muscle aches.

Note, however, that common OTC pain relievers may also prevent your body from generating the heat it needs to fight a cold or flu virus. Make sure your doctor is aware if your fever lasts for more than 3 days or is greater than 103°F. More important, before giving these products to a child, you should always consult with your pediatrician or pharmacist because of potential harmful side effects. Adults who are taking these OTC products for more than a few days should also speak with their physician to avoid any significant potential adverse side effects. Although these drugs are standard products that we all have in our medicine cabinet, they can be dangerous. Tylenol can cause liver toxicity. Aspirin can cause Reye's syndrome in children, which is characterized by fever, vomiting, and disturbances of consciousness progressing to coma and convulsions. Nonsteroidal anti-inflammatory drugs (ibuprofen) can cause gastrointestinal (GI) side effects.

- Skip the cough suppressants (e.g., dextromethorphan, codeine, hydrocodone), unless your cough is preventing you from sleeping or is so violent that you feel as if you could break a rib.

OTC cough suppressants dull your cough reflex so that you will lose the defense mechanism that is protecting your lungs from infection. Remember, coughing clears your breathing passages and prevents infection from reaching your lungs and the rest of your body. You may find it helpful to sleep with your head elevated 6–8 inches above your feet to reduce nighttime coughing.

- Drink plenty of fluids to soothe a sore throat, including hot water with lemon and honey (the honey coats your throat). Warm water gargles made with chamomile tea, fresh lemon juice, or apple cider may also offer relief.

Gargle with a warm salt water mixture made of ¼ teaspoon of salt in 8 ounces of warm water. Cough drops, hard candy, and sugarless gum can also be soothing to the throat because they stimulate the secretion of saliva, which bathes and cleanses the throat.

- Anesthetize your throat with Chloroseptic or another OTC liquid anesthetic.

However, if your throat is so sore that it is difficult to swallow, see your physician immediately to check for a bacterial infection such as strep throat. If your sore throat causes hoarseness, I recommend complete voice rest: Talking when you have an inflamed larynx may lead to more irritation and temporary loss of your voice. If you can't swallow and start drooling because you can't swallow your saliva, it is important for you to go to the nearest emergency room *immediately*.

- Humidifying the air around you with a vaporizer or humidifier, especially where you sleep, can help during the dry fall and winter months.

Adding moisture to the air prevents irritation caused by dry mucous membranes. I recommend a humidifier with a ultraviolet (UV) light, (i.e., Slant/Fin), which will kill bacteria and fungi. Warm compresses or a heating pad or lamp may be useful to relieve pain and swelling in the sinus areas. For a more direct form of adding moisture, try saline nasal sprays or saline irrigation.

- Avoid air pollutants, especially smoke-filled rooms, and fumes from household cleaners or paint.

Using Over-the-Counter Products Safely

OTC remedies are reliable and easy to obtain. However, they can be just as dangerous as prescription medications if you do not use them correctly. By following these simple rules, you can make sure that you are using OTC medicines safely:

1. Always read the labels and know the ingredients in the products you choose.

2. Make sure that the product will not interfere with any prescription or holistic medication(s) you are currently taking.

3. Never take more than the recommended dose without checking with your doctor first.

4. A true aspirin allergy is rare. However, if you know that you are allergic to aspirin, you should also avoid nonsteroidal anti-inflammatory drugs (NSAIDs) because they are chemically similar to aspirin.

5. OTC antihistamines can cause drowsiness. You should avoid driving or performing activities that require alertness when taking these medications. Infants and young children are extremely sensitive to the side effects of antihistamines and nasal decongestants: They can become irritable, restless, or drowsy. Check with your pediatrician before dosing your child with these cold or allergy products.

ACUTE RECURRENT SINUSITIS OR RHINOSINUSITIS

If either a viral or bacterial infection lasts longer than 4 weeks despite antibiotics, or if you experience at least four consecutive recurrences of acute sinusitis or rhinosinusitis, you may be diagnosed with acute recurrent sinusitis. Many of my patients can effectively treat their acute symptoms within 2 weeks, but as soon as they stop taking their medicines their initial symptoms recur. They are suffering from an acute recurrent form of sinusitis or chronic sinusitis.

This repetitive nature is actually a very common complaint among patients whose previous treatments have failed. These people experience some temporary relief, but as soon as they stop taking their medicines their condition worsens.

The cause of acute recurrent sinusitis or chronic rhinosinusitis can be one of many factors, including:

- Treatment with the wrong medicines
- Anatomical problems that lead to irreversible obstruction, which require surgery
- Continuous exposure to pollution, fungus, and environmental irritants
- Cigarette smoking or frequent contact with secondhand smoke
- Noncompliance with medicines and treatment
- Use of recreational nasal drugs (e.g., sniffing cocaine or glue)

Often, I find that patients get recurrent infections because they may have needed a 3- to 8-week course of medicines or sometimes longer, yet they took the medications only for the first 2 weeks. Or they needed 2 weeks of medicine and only took 7 or 10 days worth. The problem was simply not treated long enough to begin with. The symptoms quelled to the point at which the patients thought that they were better, but in actuality they never got rid of the root of the problem. And when they stopped their medicine, the infection flared again.

Others may be experiencing allergies, which may be a component of their chronic or acute recurrent sinusitis. It's important for your physician to determine all of the causes of your recurrent problems. It is only when each cause is properly identified that each problem can be addressed and treated appropriately. Very often, though, I find that acute recurrent sinusitis is just chronic sinusitis with recurrent bouts; therefore, the chronic underlying problem needs to be addressed.

Treating Acute Recurrent Sinusitis or Rhinosinusitis

The treatment for acute recurrent sinusitis is, in most cases, a course of antibiotics that can last for 3–8 weeks. I may recommend a course of nasal steroids to bring down excessive inflammation. I also recommend hydrating the nose with nasal saline sprays, irrigation, and steam, especially when it is dry in the winter. Hydration can break up the thick secretions. Decongestants and mucolytics can be helpful as well. You will also need to address all of the reasons causing the infection, including allergies, foods, and environmental and anatomical issues.

CHRONIC SINUSITIS OR RHINOSINUSITIS

A sinus infection lasting longer than 4 weeks should be considered more than just an acute infection and, in fact, should be considered a chronic sinus infection or chronic sinusitis. You can differentiate between an acute recurrent problem and chronic sinusitis because the symptoms of acute recurrent sinusitis will resolve after an adequate course of therapy. If 4 weeks of therapy does not yield any relief or minimal relief, then you may be suffering from a chronic problem. You may get intermittent relief because patients with chronic sinusitis typically note that their symptoms come and go, with acute exacerbations recurring to varying degrees.

According to a clinical outcome study performed at Harvard University, the chronic symptoms associated with chronic sinus disease can impair the quality of life of a sufferer more severely than heart disease impairs someone with congestive heart failure. This means that if you suffer from sinusitis, your sinus disease can be debilitating to your overall health and your lifestyle. And for those physicians and other well-intentioned folks who tell you to just live with it, this Harvard study proves that some people really have no idea just how miserable you can feel when your sinuses are out of control.

Treating Chronic Sinusitis or Rhinosinusitis

Chronic sinusitis is usually treated with a combination of medications, nasal irrigation, and débridement (endoscopic removal of infected tissue and obstructions). The therapy consists of a combination of antimicrobial, antifungal, and/or anti-inflammatory medications. The goal is to allow the sinuses to return to near-normal physiological function.

Chronic sinusitis often requires lifelong management. Just as high blood pressure can be controlled but not cured, the same holds true for chronic sinus disease. However, by following specific treatment guidelines, you can be symptom-free and comfortable. I've treated many patients with chronic sinusitis who continue to develop new infections despite good medical therapies or previous surgery. While I can usually make them feel significantly better both in the short and in the long term, their sinuses will likely become infected and inflamed again. However, with the advances being made in medicines and technology, chronic sinus sufferers can now count on major improvement in their conditions for longer periods of time. By following these treatments, most sufferers will find that they feel much better. In my practice, some of my patients have described the relief that they have obtained with chronic sinus care and management as "a new lease on life."

BIOFILMS AND CURING CHRONIC SINUSITIS

While inflammation is the direct cause of rhinosinusitis, other factors may be at work that can cause the disease to become not only chronic but difficult to permanently cure. According to a new theory, a matrix forms in the sinuses that house the fungal or bacterial infection. This matrix is called a biofilm. This biofilm anchors to the surface of the sinus and is difficult to remove. Biofilms are slimy to the touch: pond scum is an example of a biofilm found in nature. In the body, common dental plaque is considered to be a type of biofilm. The biofilms found in the sinuses appear as a yellow-green gelatinous mucus that looks like apricot jelly and/or a slimy mucus that looks like the jelly found around fish when it is refrigerated.

Biofilms have now been implicated in many infectious processes, including periodontitis, musculoskeletal infections, cystic fibrosis pneumonia, chronic sinus disease, and CAID. The latest research has begun to show that the biofilm structure creates the possibility that certain bacteria or fungi can evade antibiotic and other therapy. What's more, biofilms can deliberately release their bacteria, causing new acute infections. Unfortunately because of the biofilm properties, the only way to resolve these infections is by mechanical removal of the biofilms in the sinuses. This can occur only by irrigation and/or débridement.

Related Signs and Symptoms of Sinusitis and Rhinosinusitis

Aside from the signs and symptoms already covered, there are a few conditions that are specifically related to sinusitis and rhinosinusitis. Read through the following to determine if you are suffering from any of these issues, which can affect your overall health.

SINUS HEADACHES

Most sinus headaches are located in the cheeks, brow, and forehead and around and behind the eyes. Occasionally, headache pain may be felt on the top of the head or the back of the head. Patients may even complain that they feel strange sensations in their scalp, which can be very sensitive to touch. Pain can radiate to the temples or the teeth.

Headaches in the sinuses are typically caused by pressure changes in the sinus cavities. When the natural opening of a sinus or many sinuses are blocked by inflammation, no matter what the cause, including infection, polyps, environmental irritating substances (cigarette smoke) or allergy, a pressure gradient occurs between the inside of the sinus and the outside world. Air in the sinus is absorbed by the mucous membranes lining the sinuses. This causes a vacuum effect (negative pressure), which pulls on the lining membranes of the sinus wall, including the nerves that feed the membranes. This can cause a feeling of fullness or dull to sharp pain, as if someone were ripping the skin off your bones. Of course, the intensity depends on the individual's sensitivity and the amount of negative pressure created by the obstruction.

The pain of sinus headaches can occur in the area of the particular sinus involved. For example, the ethmoid sinuses can cause pain between the eyes or behind the eyes. If the maxillary sinuses are involved you may feel pain in your cheeks or upper teeth. However, the headache from a particular sinus can also radiate to other areas of the head. This is called "referred" pain. For instance, when inflammation of the frontal sinuses is involved you may experience pain above the eyes, in the forehead, across the bridge of the nose, or in the temples. If the sphenoid sinuses are involved, headaches can be in the center of the head or may radiate to the top or to the back of the head. You can even experience referred pain without having pain in the affected sinus area.

Sinus Headaches vs. Migraine Headache

A sinus headache can range from mild to excruciating to the point at which you can feel debilitated. A sinus headache can also spark a migraine headache. This occurs when there is pressure on the blood vessels in the sinus cavities. Many patients have sinus headaches at times and migraine headaches at other times. Or sinus headaches can turn into migraine headaches.

It is possible to tell the difference between a sinus headache and a migraine headache. Sinus headaches often occur with other sinus signs and symptoms of sinus disease; these symptoms are absent during a migraine headache, unless the migraine is sparked by the sinus headache. A migraine is usually unilateral (on one side of the head) although it may involve both sides (bilateral). A migraine headache also tends to build over time and has four unique phases.

The first phase is known as the "prodrome," which usually occurs a day before the migraine. You may either feel depressed or experience a sense of unusual well-being during this time. A migraine attack is often triggered by a period of intense activity associated with anxiety, tension, or rage. The actual migraine headache can occur at any time of the day or night but occurs frequently on waking.

The second phase is the aura. Although the aura differs for each sufferer, most people tend to repeat their aura pattern with each successive headache. Some report seeing black and white lines, like those seen by heat waves. Sometimes they experience black and white flashing lights or zigzag colored patterns with dark centers moving across their field of vision. There can be numbness of the face, arms, or feet. Others experience a loss of vision or ptosis (droopy eyelid), which can occur before the migraine. You may complain of vertigo (dizziness). As the aura disappears, you often experience a unilateral headache, which appears on the side of the head opposite to where you might have previously felt the visual aura or numbness. The transition from aura to headache may be accompanied by light sleep or a momentary loss of consciousness. The aura usually lasts for 10–40 minutes.

The actual headache pain usually starts above one eye and spreads over the entire side of the head to the back; in some cases, the pain starts in the back and moves forward. The pain spreads and intensifies to a severe throbbing, aching headache and may be worse when lying down. Shaking the head, coughing, or straining/lifting can make the headache worse. Photophobia, or extreme light sensitivity, can occur with or without nausea, vomiting, or a chill. The duration of the headache is usually between 1 and 3 hours. The recovery is the last phase of the migraine. When the attack ends, you can experience a feeling of well-being.

There are other types of headaches that people suffer from that are not clearly linked to CAID or CAID symptoms. However, I would not be surprised to find that these headaches are indeed related. What's more, it is possible to suffer from more than one form of headache at a time. We know that sinus headaches may occur simultaneously with any of these other forms. Some of these types of headaches are the following:

- Vascular headaches encompass all headache conditions, including migraines and cluster headaches, in which blood vessels swell and cause a throbbing type of pain. Vascular headaches often increase during physical exertion.
- Cluster headaches are a type of vascular headache that occur in groups over a period of time. For example, you might suffer from 4 to 10 headaches in a day. Sufferers of cluster headaches are generally affected in the spring or autumn. This type of headache is often described as a burning or piercing sensation. It may be throbbing or constant, and the scalp may be tender. These headaches are not known to be associated with CAID or allergies as of yet, but I think there may be some connection. Treatment is largely preventative: Those who suffer are often prescribed cortico-steroids or antiepileptic drugs.
- Temporomandibular joint (TMJ) pain was once thought to be caused by an arthritic change in the bottom jaw, but this type of

headache is now classified as myofascial pain dysfunction (MPD) syndrome and is thought to be caused primarily by muscular stress in the lower jaw brought on by the daily stressors of life. MPD is characterized by a dull, aching pain in and around the ear, with pain radiating to the side of the scalp, back of the head, or down the neck, and tender areas in the jaw muscles. You may also have a stabbing pain when you bite or touch the TMJ, and this can radiate to your ear. This headache is not directly caused by CAID. However, we know that there is a strong association between CAID and stress as well as dental disease. Both stress and dental disease are known causes of TMJ. Many of my patients suffer from both TMJ and sinus headaches. Treatment with drugs that prevent chronic tension-type headache is often effective, particularly tricyclic antidepressants. Your dentist may be able to make you a dental appliance and/or work on correcting your bite, which can alleviate TMJ pain, grinding, or a dental occlusion problem.

- Tension headaches are the most common form of headache and are thought to be related to muscle tightening in the back of the neck and/or scalp. They are usually described as a dull, aching, and nonpulsating pain that can affect either or both sides of the head and occur in the forehead, temples, or back of the head and/or neck. Typical symptoms for this type of headache include a tightening band-like feeling that encircles the neck and/or head that is accompanied by a gripping, "vice-like" ache. If you experience this type of headache infrequently, OTC analgesics or anti-inflammatories are good remedy choices. Meditation and exercises may be helpful. However, if you have tension headaches with any regularity, your doctor can prescribe an anti-depressant, which can help alleviate this pain whether or not you have been diagnosed with depression.

Recounting Painful Headache Experiences

Some of my patients tell me that they can't lift their head off the pillow when they experience either migraines or sinus headaches. For instance, my patient Matthew came to see me when his headaches became so bad that he couldn't function at work. A 43-year-old executive, Matthew's headaches continually disrupted his sleep, preventing him from performing properly at work. When he awoke, he found himself so congested that he couldn't breathe. Matthew had been to allergists, neurologists, and internists and had taken "a million medicines," all without success. He was told that he was experiencing migraines; a condition surgery could not cure. His migraines were treated with various medicines, but to no avail. The pain would become so intense that it felt as if someone were sticking an ice pick into his forehead. He would often be awakened by these headaches. To add insult to injury, Matthew also suffered from constant acid reflux, which worsened when he became congested.

I did a complete workup on Matthew and found his migraines had been misdiagnosed: Matthew was suffering from sinus headaches caused by the swelling and closure of the nasal passageways. I performed sinus surgery to open his passageways, which alleviated his headaches immediately. I put Matthew on a maintenance program of traditional medicines and holistic care to control his sinuses. I treated his acid reflux with various medicines. After his sinus surgery Matthew reported that his reflux no longer bothered him except on a rare occasion, usually related to his diet. He is now able to sleep at night. Although he continues treatment for his sinus disease, he is no longer debilitated and is functioning quite well at work.

Sinus Headache Treatments

The first step to breaking the cycle of sinus headaches is to clear up and control your sinus problems. At this point, you might see your headaches disappear or improve significantly. Some of my patients have also found relief by eliminating caffeine, chocolate, and other stimulants from their diet.

Yet sometimes in the face of only mild sinus symptoms, patients will still complain of terrible sinus headaches. These patients may even have a negative computed tomography (CT) scan (a CT scan that appears normal), but the endoscopic examination will show a narrowing of the passageways, or more often, very reactive membranes (membranes that might look normal but swell significantly when exposed to particles that you may be sensitive to). Unfortunately, because these patients often have a normal CT scan, they usually end up seeing many different physicians before they are correctly diagnosed. This is a very difficult diagnosis to make because patients may appear normal in between bouts or even during the later part of the headache when the swelling resolves. Furthermore, these patients are most often treated successfully with medicines; surgery may be required, but rarely. When surgery is required, patients typically find great relief.

For example, Claire was a 28–year–old woman who came to me complaining of bad sinus headaches that occurred in her forehead, cheeks, and teeth. She had been suffering from these headaches for years, probably since the time she began to menstruate when she was a teenager. Claire had been to many different physicians, each of whom could not find anything wrong with her because her CT scans were normal. Allergy testing showed that she had mild allergies, but nothing significant enough to produce these types of reactions. Claire told me that she has always been sensitive to cigarette smoke, car exhaust, and perfumes. She realized that when she was around these odors, her headaches flared.

I first examined her sinuses, and they appeared to look fairly normal. But when I was able to examine Claire immediately after she was exposed to one of her known irritants, she instantly began to flare. I noticed that even touching the inside of her nose with an endoscope caused a reaction. I knew that it was her reactive nature that brought on her headaches and congestion.

For treatment, I put Claire on a topical nasal steroid spray as well as a decongestant and antihistamine for her allergies. These medications brought some resolution to her other CAID symptoms, but her headaches did not go away. Together, we decided that I should perform functional endoscopic sinus surgery (FESS). Today, Claire is headache-free.

NASAL POLYPS

Nasal polyps are small growths that occur in the nasal cavities. They can be as small as the tip of a ballpoint pen or as large as a grape. Even small polyps can obstruct sinus openings, which can allow sinusitis to develop. Polyps are diagnosed via a CT scan and/or endoscopy.

Polyps are caused by inflammation. Some physicians and scientists believe that polyps result from allergies, infection, or exposure to smoke or other pollutants, such as household chemicals or dust. Recent research has confirmed that polyps are instead caused only by infections. The other causes inflame the membranes, which results in thickened mucus, which then causes infection. The infection then causes the polyps to grow. Once polyps form, they can block the sinus openings and trigger more inflammation—which can lead to even more polyps. Furthermore, the obstruction caused by polyps leads to nasal airway blockage. When polyps grow around the olfactory nerve, your sense of smell, and subsequently taste, can diminish or disappear.

Treating Nasal Polyps

To reduce the size of nasal polyps so that breathing can return to normal, you must break the inflammatory cycle. Polyps may need to be removed surgically. However, they tend to recur, so medication still must be taken to control them even after they are removed. I often prescribe nasal steroid sprays or oral steroids, such as prednisone, to reduce inflammation. Antibiotics and/or antifungals (oral or topical) are also used to eliminate any underlying infection. If you have allergies, antihistamines may help.

Polyps that are obstructive and can trigger sinusitis may need to be surgically removed. This outpatient procedure can be performed with local anesthesia (see Chapter 12).

DEVIATED SEPTUM

If the wall between your nostrils (the septum) is crooked because of an injury or anatomical abnormality, it can create air turbulence that can irritate the sinus membranes. This irritation can cause swelling, which will impede normal sinus drainage. A septal deviation can also create significant nasal obstruction, enough to cause difficulty breathing through your nose, loud snoring or sleep apnea, and/or mouth breathing.

Obstructed sinuses will further compound the problems. I believe that normal nasal flow is necessary for proper mucociliary flow. When the nasal cavities are obstructed by a septal deviation or turbinate hypertrophy, there will be abnormal mucus flow with crusting and infection. Infection can cause more swelling in the nose and sinuses, leading to further obstruction and creating a vicious cycle.

If you have been told that you have a deviated septum, it's very important that you try to prevent recurring or chronic sinusitis by taking steps to reduce nasal congestion. I always tell my patients who have a deviated septum to frequently irrigate or wash their nose with OTC, prescription, or premixed saline nasal spray. By keeping your nasal passages clear and moist, you can help reduce congestion and promote sinus drainage.

Decoding My Problem

The first step to better health is to review your results from Part One of the CAID Quiz (p. 70–71). Locate your score so that you can define your next course of action. Follow these guidelines:

- If your score is between 0 and 10, you can treat your symptoms with OTC medications for the first 48 hours. If the symptoms persist, see your primary-care physician.
- If your score is between 11 and 40, then you need to see your primary-care physician immediately.
- If your score is between 41 and 80, you need to see an ear, nose, and throat (ENT) specialist.
- If your score is 80 or more, you need to see an ENT who specializes in treating CAID or at least in treating sinusitis, allergies, and/or asthma.

Next, read the following sections about treatments. Based on your score, you can decide on a course of action. Follow the recommendations for one complete month, and then take the quiz again. If your score does not improve after following your treatment, go to the next level of care. Your physician can recommend an ENT (otolaryngologist) who he or she feels comfortable working with. Your doctor may also recommend another type of specialist, or practioner, if necessary. Make sure that all of the practitioners who treat you communicate with each other. This is paramount in providing you with the best results possible.

I treat my patients with any level of sinus disease with various medicines in addition to antibiotics. I often use medicines in combination, depending on each patient's unique clinical picture. Your treatment options will be based on your complete medical history, physical examination, and test results. Based on these findings your doctor will be able to prescribe a treatment plan that will work for you.

TREATMENT OPTIONS

Currently, there are new medicines and successful combinations of traditional and holistic care that can treat sinus disease. The sinus problems of the vast majority of sinus disease sufferers can be successfully treated with medication alone. This may include a combination of nasal sprays, decongestants, antihistamines, antibiotics, and antifungals. But before we talk about prescription medications, there is one home remedy that I recommend to all of my patients: nasal irrigation. This process is the first step in my five-step plan for complete sinus health.

Irrigating the Sinuses

Using a mild nasal saline spray to regularly cleanse and moisturize the sinuses is probably the best thing you can do for your health. Saline sprays are OTC remedies that are made by many different companies. You should experiment with the different formulations and see which one agrees with you best. Saline spray works well when patients have an acute infection.

A nebulizer will work the same way, but I usually recommend buying a nebulizer only for the administration of prescription topical preparations because a spray bottle is much cheaper and that is all you really need to place mist in your nose. However, a nebulizer gives great relief: It feels like going into a mini steam room and is very soothing.

Preparing for Irrigation

If you have recurrent or chronic sinus disease, you may require more aggressive therapy with saline solution. You will need to irrigate with a neti pot (i.e., Baraka pot) or an irrigation device (i.e., Hydro Pulse). You can purchase a neti pot at most pharmacies or health-food stores, and irrigation devices can be found at most pharmacies. Some people use a simple squeeze bottle, but the drawback is the reflux of infection that can reenter a squeeze bottle. I prefer that my patients use the neti pot or an irrigation device. A squeeze bottle that does not reflux would be a good choice, but the neti pot and the irrigation devices seem to have a more steady flow of saline delivered with more reliable pressure.

I usually recommend that patients irrigate with a solution that has the same amount of salt that is contained in our bodies. This is called "normal saline" or "isotonic saline." Some doctors sell and recommend hypertonic solutions, which contain a higher concentration of salt than that of our bodies. Others recommend hypotonic solutions, which contain less salt than that of our bodies. But I usually recommend normal saline solution to start because it is the most well tolerated and least inflammatory.

You can buy prepared sterile saline from most pharmacies, but large quantities may require a prescription from your doctor. Some insurance companies will cover this as it is a necessary treatment for the care of your sinuses. However, if your insurance won't pay for it, you can inexpensively and easily make the saline yourself. The drawback is that it is time-consuming to make saline the right way, and you really want to be exact when you whip up a batch of normal saline.

If you decide make your own solution, start with distilled water; your tap water may contain impurities that can cause inflammation of your sinuses. Bring distilled water to a boil. Carefully and accurately measure 8 ounces of the hot water. Add ¼ teaspoon of salt to the water, and let the mixture cool to room temperature. For a larger quantity, use 4 teaspoons of salt to 1 gallon of water. Be sure to measure accurately; too much or too little salt can damage the mucus-producing cells and hair cells in the nose. Congratulations, you have successfully made normal saline that has no preservatives.

Some people like to irrigate with room-temperature saline, others like warm saline, and others like saline that is cool or slightly below room temperature. Try all three and see which makes you feel best. Remember that you should not put saline that is too hot or too cold into your nose and sinuses, because you can burn or damage the inside of your nose.

Using a Neti Pot A neti pot is an ancient Indian tool used to cleanse the nose. Choose a neti pot with a tapered conical tip at the spout end that is the right size for your nostrils. Fill the pot with the cooled saline (Diagram 16a).

Tilt your head to one side, and gently insert the spout of the neti pot into the raised, upper nostril (Diagram 16b). Continue to breathe through your mouth, and slowly pour the saline into your upper nostril.

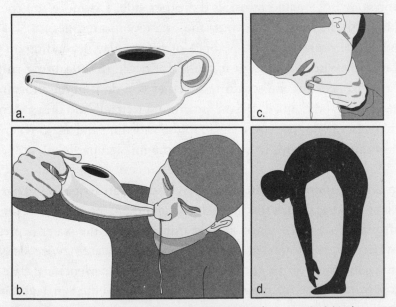

Diagram 16 a: A neti pot. b: Inserting the neti pot into the nose. c: Draining the saline solution from the sinuses. d: Toe touches complete the draining process.

The saline should pour through the upper nostril and out the other (lower) nostril into the sink (you can also try this in the shower). If the saline drains out of your mouth, lower your forehead toward your chin. Keep breathing through your mouth and relax: the saline should gently flow through the nose. Raise the neti pot slowly to create a steady flow of saline solution through the upper nostril and out the lower nostril (Diagram 16c). When you're done, compress one nostril at a time by placing pressure on it with your finger and then blow your other nostril out by exhaling firmly several times to clear the nasal passages. Then reverse the tilt of your head and repeat the process on the other side by pouring saline into the other nostril.

When you are finished irrigating, you should stretch and do toe touches for 2 minutes (Diagram 16d). When you are as far flexed as you can be with the top of your head pointing at the floor, turn your head to the left, then to the right. Prepare yourself before you stand up: The saline may pour out of your nose, even though you may have thought that it had all drained while you were blowing. Repeat blowing each side of your nose while pressing the other side. Do more toe touches and then stand up and drain your sinuses a few more times.

Nasal irrigation can be done once or twice a day, depending on your level of congestion. Although it sounds difficult, this cleansing ritual is very easy to perform and soothing whether you do it in the morning or in the evening before bed. If you are around irritants and dust at work, I highly recommend that you irrigate in the morning and again when you return home from work to wash out all the inhaled particles.

Using an Irrigation Apparatus You can also try an irrigation apparatus. This is an electric device that is used in much the same manner as the neti pot. It provides a more aggressive cleansing because the water is pressurized. The irrigation apparatus should be used once or twice daily for chronic conditions or more often when you are experiencing a flare-up.

I personally use an irrigation apparatus. I feel that in bad cases it breaks the infection up better than a neti pot. A neti pot is, however, enough for mild cases of infection. Use the irrigation device the same way you use the neti pot. After irrigating with the irrigation apparatus,

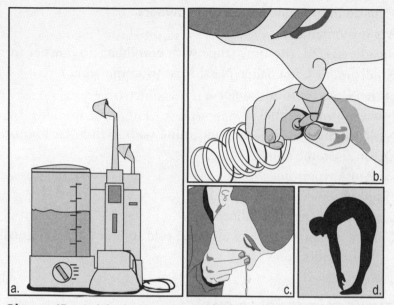

Diagram 17 a: An irrigation apparatus provides a more aggressive cleaning than the neti pot. b: Inserting the tip of the irrigator into the nose. c: Draining the saline solution from the sinuses. d: Toe touches complete the draining process.

you should do the same toe touching exercises that I described for the neti pot so that the saline completely drains from your sinuses (Diagram 17). You can get an irrigation device in certain pharmacies or via the Internet.

The saline solution used during irrigation will not always get past the blockages and will not enter the most remote cells. In addition, it will seep into some of the cells and get caught there, only to result in potential streams of water dripping from your nose later in the day. Unfortunately, this usually occurs at the most inopportune times, like when you are out on a romantic evening or when you are talking to your boss. This is nothing to worry about except that it might be a little embarrassing. Nevertheless, the way to avoid this is to stretch and place your head in different directions after irrigating, thereby completely draining your sinuses.

Over-the-Counter Saline Sprays and Powders
Ayr (isotonic saline)
BreatheseaseXL (isotonic saline with emollients in powder form)
Goldberger's Ultra Saline Nasal Mist (isotonic saline)
Little Noses (isotonic saline)
Nasal (isotonic saline)
NeilMed Sinus Relief (isotonic saline with sodium bicarbonate)
Ocean (isotonic saline)
SaltAire (hypertonic saline)
Simply Saline (isotonic saline)
SinuCleanse (isotonic saline)
Generic products (sodium chloride sold in liter bottles is usually by
prescription only)

MASTERING ROUTINE NOSE BLOWING

For anyone with any form of sinusitis, it's important to keep your nose clear by frequent blowing. However, some doctors believe that blowing your nose too forcefully can actually be detrimental: It can force the mucus, and any germs it contains, into the sinus cavities. Others believe that this is not true.

I believe that the correct way to blow your nose is to clear one nostril at a time by pressing one side closed, then blowing. Next, do the same on the other side. Afterward, inhale deeply through your nose forcing any excess mucus into the back of your nose and down your throat, where you can swallow it or spit it out. Most people don't like to do this, but it won't hurt you and does help prevent further sinusitis. Remember, all day long the healthy nose makes 1–2 liters of mucus, which traps particles in the nose and then it passes into your throat and you swallow it. Sniffing in does the same thing.

YOUR MOTHER WAS WRONG

I have never met a person who has not picked his or her nose sometime in the past. Although picking our nose is taboo in today's society and considered disgusting, people pick their noses to remove infected crusting that is irritating them or to remove scabbing as a result of nasal dryness and bleeding. These crusts and scabs are blocking your breathing, making you uncomfortable. So it is good to get them out. The best way to do it is with a tissue or to blow it out.

From a medical point of view, the worst part about picking your nose is putting your dirty fingers into your otherwise clean nose. So my first suggestion is that you wash your hands before you pick your nose. In light of current etiquette, others do not want to watch you do this, so you should probably do it in private. Using a tissue over your finger is also probably a good idea.

If you are frequently plagued by the need to remove stuff from your nose, you might want to try a nasal spray and/or antibiotic ointment like Neosporin, Bactroban, or Bacitracin to soften up the chronic crusts and scabs. Apply it with a tissue or a cotton swab. Wait a few minutes and then try to blow it out. If you remove a scab, it will probably bleed again. The best treatment for this is to apply ointment to the site after removing the scab, which will decrease the new scab formation. It will also keep it clean. Reapplication of the ointment will keep the scab soft and allow it to heal quickly.

Often, I will meet concerned parents who are worried about their child picking his or her nose. I explain that their child is doing what most adults do, but without proper hygiene. They should teach their children to wrap a tissue around their finger before they insert it into their nose. Using a vaporizer or humidifier in the winter will help reduce crusting and scabbing, which will reduce their need to pick their nose. Lastly, most children can apply ointment or spray their nose with saline, both of which can soften crusts and scabs. Many children successfully irrigate with a neti pot or a nasal irrigator.

PRESCRIPTION MEDICINES

Don't Be Afraid to Take Medication

Patients very often come into my office afraid to take medication. Their fears are usually based on inaccurate information that they have been given regarding medicines. You should understand that despite the fact that every medicine has its risks, when taken properly most medication will help rather than hurt you. For example, I had a patient who came to me many years ago. During the initial consultation, Stella told me that she usually had a few stiff drinks (three or four and sometimes more) each night and an assortment of wine and beer through the day. She smoked two packs of cigarettes a day and confessed that she often played around with recreational drugs, including marijuana and cocaine. Yet for all the abuse her body took, Stella was able to hold a job successfully as an executive at a major firm.

Stella came to see me because she felt sick all the time and had difficulty breathing. I quickly realized that she was suffering from a bad sinus infection. She had also created a large hole in her nose from her cocaine use. After diagnosing her chronic sinus problem, I told her that she needed to be put on antibiotics for at least 8 weeks, and that I would also start her on nasal and oral steroids. Stella's response to this was simply: "But aren't antibiotics and steroids dangerous?" I had to laugh: The medications I was prescribing would not harm her, unlike the drugs, alcohol, and cigarettes she didn't seem to worry about using every day. This example is extreme, but all of the medicines that I prescribe have been tested in clinical trials before they get U.S. Food and Drug Administration (FDA) approval.

Keep Your Treatment Goals Realistic

It's important to set achievable treatment goals, and to remain patient during the healing process. The expectation that a single 10-day course of antibiotics will magically cure you is unrealistic, especially because your chronic sinusitis or rhinosinusitis may have been with you for several years. Therefore, it is important to follow your doctor's specific recommendations to provide you with the chance for a complete recovery or at least maximum improvement.

ANTIBIOTICS

Antibiotics are prescription medications produced by or derived from certain fungi or plants that can destroy or inhibit the growth of other microorganisms, called bacteria. Antibiotics are widely used to prevent and treat infectious diseases. Antibiotics are prescribed when your body has been inundated with several types of unwanted bacteria. The antibiotic chosen by your physician will not kill all bacteria living in your body, but will kill most of the unwanted bacteria, so that your body can fight off the rest. They give your immune system a helping hand in killing the bacteria that do not belong in your body.

I believe that antibiotics are wonderful, effective medications that help our bodies fight infections. Antibiotics have saved millions of lives since they were first developed. Furthermore, they have made the lives of tens of millions more comfortable. In the pre-antibiotic era, it was common for people to die of sinus infections, bronchitis, and pneumonia. Today, through the proper use of antibiotics, these deaths are rare.

When Should I Take Antibiotics?

You may be prescribed antibiotics when there is a confirmed diagnosis of a bacterial infection manifesting as acute, recurrent, or chronic sinusitis or rhinitis. Typically, patients who complain of yellow, green, or brown nasal discharge or postnasal drip have a bacterial infection.

First and foremost: Take all of the antibiotics as directed. Do not skip any doses as this can lead to resistant bacteria, as well as recurring symptoms. Even though you will probably begin to feel better within the first few days of taking an antibiotic, the treatment of a bacterial infection causing chronic sinusitis or rhinosinusitis requires a minimum of 3–8 weeks of antibiotics. You are not doing yourself any favors by saving half the prescription for the next bacterial infection.

Who Should Not Take Antibiotics?

There are people who are allergic to particular classes of antibiotics. The most common is the penicillin family. When you are allergic to a medication, it means that you can't take the whole class of medication. However, you need to be careful when determining if you are truly allergic to the medication. For example, some people develop a stomachache after taking Amoxil; this does not mean that they are allergic to Amoxil or penicillin. When taking antibiotics, keep careful records on how each class of antibiotics has affected you. Then you can talk with your physician about safely prescribing the one with the least negative side effects.

Risks and Side Effects of Antibiotics

Antibiotics not only kill the bacteria causing your sinus infection but also kill the friendly bacteria that line your intestines. These bacteria normally help with digestion, and by eliminating them, you can give yourself an unexpected bout of antibiotic-induced diarrhea. Here are a few things you can take to minimize this uncomfortable side effect:

- Acidophilus is a probiotic available as a pill or powder of the normal bacterial flora of the intestines. Taking this during a course of antibiotics and continuing for 2 weeks thereafter can help prevent diarrhea and yeast infections. I strongly suggest that you take this if you are going to be on antibiotics for longer than 2 weeks or if you have had previous diarrhea or fungal infections from antibiotics in the past. There are other probiotics that you can take if you have a sensitive stomach; your physician or health-care practitioner can recommend what is best for you.
- Ask your doctor to prescribe a more intestine-friendly antibiotic. Although this is not a guarantee because people react differently to various antibiotics.
- Stop the antibiotic if the diarrhea is severe, if your stool is bloody, or if you have severe stomach cramps or vomiting. Contact your doctor immediately.

Vomiting can occur after a dose of the antibiotics. If this happens, stop taking the antibiotic and contact your doctor. It probably won't happen again as this reaction is very uncommon. However, you and your doctor should decide the best course of action if this happens. You may need a different antibiotic. This is probably not an allergy.

A rash can also occur during antibiotic use. This may be due to an allergy to the antibiotic. If you develop a rash, stop taking the antibiotic immediately until you contact your doctor. Your doctor will probably suggest that you take a dose of Benadryl, an antihistamine that can temporarily decrease an allergic rash and itching. A rash usually does not warrant a trip to the emergency room, but you should call your doctor immediately to let him or her know. However, you should immediately see your doctor or go to the emergency room if you have one or more of the following signs of a severe allergic reaction:

- Wheezing
- Difficulty breathing (not just nasal congestion)
- Difficulty swallowing due to a tight throat
- Excessive drooling with difficulty swallowing
- Swollen joints

Should I Take Probiotics?

Even if you are not suffering from diarrhea, it is a good idea to take OTC probiotics, such as acidophilus, lactobacillus, or saccharomyces boulardii lyo to preserve the normal flora in the stomach and the GI tract while on antibiotics. It is common to develop fungal infections of the nails, jock itch, or vaginal yeast infections while taking antibiotics. Fungus can also grow in any skin creases (e.g., under the breasts, in the arm pits, or in stomach rolls). Taking probiotics as well as keeping these areas dry can help prevent fungal infections from occurring. Another less common side effect is oral thrush, which can occur when antibiotics kill the normal mouth flora and allow yeast to grow inside the mouth. When this happens, you will see white patches growing on the insides of the cheeks, on the tongue, under the lips, or on the gums. Acidophilus will also help prevent thrush during antibiotic use.

Antibiotic Resistance: Reality or Myth?

There is a large and, unfortunately, growing misconception that people become resistant to antibiotics. In truth, people don't become resistant to antibiotics, the bacteria do. What's more, bacteria become resistant only when we do not take antibiotics properly. For example, when you have a bacterial infection, you are bombarded with millions of bacteria, yet only half are sensitive to a particular antibiotic, while the other half are resistant. Your body can kill off the resistant bacteria if it is helped by the antibiotic over a course of 14 days because the antibiotic is meant to kill off the sensitive bacteria. While you may start to feel better by day 7, all of the bacteria have not been killed, including the resistant bacteria. You might decide to stop the antibiotics anyway, thinking that you are well. However, the resistant bacteria can start to multiply to numbers that will make you sick again. Now you have developed a new or recurrent infection for which your antibiotic won't work. Your body will not be able to fight off this many bacteria on it's own without help of the antibiotic. And the antibiotic won't work. If you had continued to take the antibiotic the first time long enough for it to kill off all of the sensitive bacteria, your body would have killed the few resistant bacteria and you would have been cured. This is why it is important to take the complete course of antibiotics.

If you suffer from chronic sinus infections, don't worry about developing a resistance to antibiotics. These medications can be prescribed as part of a targeted treatment program that, if needed, can be used round after round until your infection has completely cleared. It is well known that antibiotic resistance can be prevented if a careful and strict approach to care is followed. This care begins with knowing which specific bacteria are causing each infection and which antibiotics are effective against that bacteria. Furthermore, your doctor is assuming that you will be compliant, taking all of your medicines without skipping any of the doses.

Others are concerned that antibiotics are dangerous. This cannot be further from the truth. Instead, it is the misuse of antibiotics that is dangerous: especially for those who do not finish their dosage or self-medicate infections with leftover pills from previous infections. These scenarios can cause the antibiotics to work improperly.

I once treated Philip, a 41-year-old man who thought he needed sinus surgery. Philip came to me complaining of repeated severe frontal headaches and constant sinus infections. He had postnasal drip with hoarseness, and a constant cough and often got laryngitis. His sense of smell and taste had diminished. Philip spent a significant amount of time in airplanes, and complained that his headaches were especially bad when he flew: His ears would get clogged and the pain in his ears and sinuses frustrated him to the point that it was making flying almost unbearable.

Philip was told by his primary-care physician that he might need sinus surgery and came to my office for a consultation. Instead of surgery, I started him on medication. I treated him with nasal steroids, antihistamines, antibiotics, and natural acidophilus. At first, Philip was reluctant to take antibiotics, but after I explained how the antibiotics worked, he decided to take them to treat the bacterial infection. With this treatment, Philip was able to avoid surgery. Best of all, he no longer has sinus headaches or sinus infections. He still flies frequently and reports that he no longer has ear pain or frontal headaches.

How Does My Physician Choose Which Oral Antibiotic to Prescribe?

It may seem like an easy decision to prescribe an antibiotic, but it is actually a complex process. I consider each patient's particular needs, allergies, previous antibiotic tolerance profile, compliance, other medicines that he is taking, severity of his sinus disease, the type of bacterial infection I am treating, and any cultures that may have been taken. Even then, the antibiotic may not work or may only partially work in helping clear his sinus infection. Luckily, there is usually more than one right choice. I have had patients who report that they went to two physicians and each gave them a different antibiotic. Well, they both may have been good choices.

Speak with your physician about all of these concerns and be sure to keep a good history of the antibiotics that you have taken. This should include all of the following:

- A list of the antibiotics to which you have had a true allergic reaction, along with the description of the allergic reaction (e.g., rash, hives, breathing difficulty, or anaphylactic reaction).
- A list of all antibiotics to which you have had other untoward responses or reactions (e.g., diarrhea, constipation, stomach upset, vaginal or other fungal infection, metal taste, joint pain, or dizziness). Your physician may tell you that a previous reaction of this

type may not necessarily repeat itself even though it may have been severe in the past.

Bacteria

The sinuses provide a good place for any bacteria to grow. Recent studies have identified both aerobic and anaerobic organisms and fungi growing within the sinuses. This makes the choice of picking an antibiotic difficult, and you may find that your physician wants to put you on more than one antibiotic during a single course of treatment. Although complicated, this is a correct choice if your doctor believes that your infection is being caused by multiple types of bacteria. The most common bacteria that cause sinusitis are *Streptococcus pneumoniae*, *Haemophilus influenzae*, and *Moraxella catarrhalis*. Others include *Staphylococcus aureus* and *Pseudomonas aeruginosa*, which often cause the more aggressive infections.

There has been a concern in recent years that there is an increased resistance in *H. influenzae* strains (54 percent resistant to Ampicillin), and *M. catarrhalis* (74 percent resistant to Ampicillin). It also appears that there is increasing resistance of *Streptococcus pneumoniae* to various antibiotics. Methicillin-resistant *Staphylococcus aureus* and *P. aeruginosa* tend to cause more aggressive infections and are harder to resolve.

Available Antibiotics

Often, the first choices for treating CAID symptoms are amoxicillin, trimethoprim-sulfamethoxazole, and erythromycin. As bacteria become more resistant to certain antibiotics, physicians are tending to choose newer versions over old standbys. The circulating bacteria usually have not had time to develop resistance to these newer antibiotics, so they may be more effective. However, the older antibiotics may still be effective, and in many cases are less expensive than the newer antibiotics. The following sections discuss the types of antibiotics used to treat CAID.

Beta-Lactams The beta-lactam antibiotics share common chemical features and include penicillins and cephalosporins. Their primary action is to interfere with the cell walls of the bacteria that are causing your infection.

Penicillins The most widely prescribed antibiotic for sinusitis has been amoxicillin (Amoxil, Polymox, Trimox, or any generic formulation). Amoxicillin is inexpensive and at one time was highly effective against the *Streptococcus pneumoniae* bacteria. However, bacterial resistance to amoxicillin has increased significantly, both among *Streptococcus pneumoniae* and *H. influenzae*. Amoxicillin-clavulanate (Augmentin) is known as augmented penicillin and is often used. Augmentin works against a wide spectrum of bacteria and is more effective against resistant strains than amoxicillin alone because the clavulanate strengthens the amoxicillin.

Ampicillin is another form of penicillin. It is an inexpensive alternative to amoxicillin but requires more doses and has more severe gastrointestinal side effects than amoxicillin. There is significant resistance to ampicillin. Dicloxacillin is a penicillin that can be used if there is an abscess in the sinus because it is effective against *Staphylococcus aureus*. UniSyn is available for intravenous use for more severe cases.

Cephalosporins These broad-spectrum antibiotics are used against *Streptococcus pneumoniae* and some are effective against *H. influenzae*. They are often classed by "generation."

- First-generation agents include cephalexin (Keflex), cefadroxil (Duricef), and cefaclor (Ceclor).
- Second- and third-generation drugs include cefuroxime (Ceftin), cefprozil (Cefzil), cefpodoxime (Vantin), loracarbef (Lorabid), cefixime (Suprax), and ceftibuten (Cidex). These are effective against a wide spectrum of bacteria and are increasingly used for respiratory infections. There are *Streptococcus pneumoniae* bacteria that are resistant to cephalosporins. Rocephin is a third-generation cephalosporin that is available only for intravenous use.

Macrolides and Azalides Macrolides and azalides are antibiotics used for bacterial sinusitis. They are effective for those allergic to penicillin as well as those who have mild to moderate symptoms. They may also be appropriate if you have taken antibiotics within 4 weeks. They work by interfering with the genetics of the bacteria. They include erythromycin, azithromycin (Zithromax) and clarithromycin (Biaxin). These antibiotics are effective against *Streptococcus pneumoniae* and *M. catarrhalis*. All but erythromycin are effective against *H. influenzae*. Clarithromycin has anti-inflammatory actions, making it a particularly good choice for treating chronic sinusitis. A new once-a-day formulation (Biaxin XL) is also available.

Trimethoprim-Sulfamethoxazole Trimethoprim–sulfamethoxazole (Bactrim, Septra, Pediazole) is also a first-line antibiotic for sinusitis. It is less expensive than amoxicillin and particularly useful if you are suffering from mild sinusitis or are allergic to penicillin. There are resistant streptococcal strains. It should not be used if you are allergic to sulfa drugs, iodine, or shellfish. A rare reaction called Stevens Johnson syndrome can occur, which can be life threatening. This antibiotic is prescribed for both adults and children.

Fluoroquinolones Fluoroquinolones (also known as quinolones) prevent bacteria from multiplying because they interfere with the bacteria's genetic material. The first quinolone used was ciprofloxacin (Cipro). Since that time other quinolones were developed, including levofloxacin (Levaquin), gemifloxacin (Factive), moxifloxacin (Avelox), and ofloxacin (Floxin). The newer fluoroquinolones are currently the most effective agents against the common bacteria that cause sinusitis. Levofloxacin was the first drug approved specifically for penicillin-resistant *Streptococcus pneumoniae*, although studies are now finding resistance to this agent as well. These agents are recommended for adults with moderate sinusitis who have already been treated with antibiotics within 6 weeks or who are allergic to beta-lactam antibiotics.

Lincosamide Lincosamides also prevent bacteria from reproducing. The most common lincosamide is clindamycin (Cleocin). This antibiotic is useful against many *Streptococcus pneumoniae* bacteria but not against *H. influenzae.* It is also effective against anaerobic organisms that cause sinusitis. One common side effect is diarrhea.

Tetracyclines Tetracyclines inhibit bacterial growth. They include doxycycline, tetracycline, and minocycline. They can be effective against *Streptococcus pneumoniae* and *M. catarrhalis*, but bacteria that are resistant to penicillin are also often resistant to doxycycline. Tetracyclines have unique side effects among antibiotics, including skin reactions to sunlight, possible burning in the throat, and stained teeth. These antibiotics should not be given to children before their adult teeth are fully present, to prevent dental staining.

Ketolides Telithromycin (Ketek) is the first antibiotic in the ketolide class. It is showing great promise in treating many of the otherwise antibiotic-resistant bacterial strains and has now been approved for treating community-acquired pneumonia (CAP), chronic obstructive lung disease, and sinusitis. It has potential liver toxicity.

Vancomycin Vancomycin (Vancocin) works well for methicillin-resistant *Staphylococcus aureus* (MRSA) infections.

How Should I Be Taking Antibiotics?

Antibiotics can be administered in different ways. The most common way to prescribe an antibiotic is orally. But in patients with recurring disease, there are many physicians who give antibiotics intravenously as an outpatient procedure. Antibiotics can also be administered topically via nebulizer, spray, or irrigation preparations. In my experience, topical antibiotics work best in patients who have already undergone sinus surgery. In patients who have not had surgery, the areas to which such antibiotics need to be applied are either partially or totally inaccessible. The bacteria in those areas will thus get suboptimal treatment and are more likely to develop resistance.

Some oral antibiotics deliver the same concentration of drug that their intravenous forms are able to provide. However, this is not true for all antibiotics. Many physicians still believe, and they may be correct, that intravenous antibiotics always deliver a more reliable drug dose. Regardless of how the antibiotic is taken, the appropriate drug concentration needs to be reached in the bloodstream to achieve results. In any case, I generally use intravenous antibiotics when:

- The patient experiences stomach upset when taking oral antibiotics
- Higher blood levels than can be achieved with the oral antibiotic are desired
- The bacterial infection is not responding to oral antibiotics despite culture sensitivity
- When the patient suffers from a complication of the sinus infection, including periorbital infection (swelling around the eye, or cellulitis), bulging eyes (proptosis), meningitis, or an eye or brain abscess
- Surgery reveals significant infection in the underlying bone of the sinuses

When Should I Use Topical Antibiotics?
There are different methods for applying antibiotics topically to the nose and sinuses:

- Nebulizer therapy
- Irrigation therapy
- Ointment

Patients who have already undergone FESS may continue to suffer from chronic or recurrent sinusitis. For these patients, it is often more effective to get the antibiotic directly on the inflamed area, instead of ingesting the medication. Most important, topical antibiotics offer the opportunity to use medications that are well tolerated topically, yet would have significant risks if ingested.

A nasal nebulizer delivers compounded medications that are aerosolized to a particle size small enough to disperse within the sinus cavities yet large enough to be deposited in the sinuses. Nasal nebulizers can be used to deliver antibiotics, antifungals, and steroids to the sinus mucus membrane. A popular nasal nebulizer is the SinuNEB System.

Side effects of medications in nebulized forms of antibiotics appear to be milder in some patients than those experienced from oral and intravenous forms. In some patients, sore throat may develop, which can be improved by gargling after each treatment. Cough may occur in patients who have asthma, which should improve with a temporary increase in the use of pulmonary inhalers. Joint pain may be observed in patients undergoing fluoroquinolone therapy. Tinnitus and hearing loss could occur with gentamicin therapy. With topical administration of antibiotics, the risk of these side effects is significantly decreased compared with oral or intravenous administration.

Nebulized Antibiotics

Ceftazidime	Levofloxacin
Cefuroxime	Ofloxacin
Ciprofloxacin	Tobramycin
Gentamicin	Vancomycin

Irrigation Antibiotic Therapy

Any of the antibiotics just listed can be added to irrigation solution, which can be administered via a neti pot or nasal irrigator. Make sure that your doctor or pharmacist gives you complete instructions on how to mix the antibiotic with the saline solution or other solution, and what special precautions need to be followed. Be sure to practice using the neti pot or nasal irrigator with regular saline solution before adding the antibiotic treatment.

Antibiotic Ointment

An OTC triple-antibiotic ointment can be used in the nose. As you breathe, this type of ointment finds its way through your sinuses and can help when you develop dry crust in your nose. Use a cotton swab to gently insert the ointment in the nose. If you feel pain or have a problem, speak with your physician.

CORTICOSTEROID MEDICATIONS

The main role of corticosteroid medications is to control inflammation. Steroid medications are chemically similar to many of your body's naturally produced hormones. These medications work by mimicking the cortisone and hydrocortisone steroids that are made by the adrenal gland. When you take these medications, you are exceeding the natural levels of steroids found in your body. This extra boost of steroids in the body helps prevent and suppress inflammation.

The decision as to whether to place a patient on topical nasal steroid sprays only or to add oral steroids depends on the severity of the inflammation. I typically prescribe nasal steroid sprays to my patients who have an inflammatory response within the nose and/or sinuses. I prescribe oral steroids when I believe that the inflammation in the sinuses is more than that which can be handled by topical steroids alone. If you suffer from nasal polyps and/or asthma and your sinuses are flaring, you are a good candidate for oral steroids because they will reduce the severe inflammation that causes these conditions. Treatment will not cure these problems but will bring them under control. Last, I may prescribe pulmonary steroid sprays to control asthma or asthmatic bronchitis. I usually place my patients on a low, short-term dose. I place those who are badly infected on higher dose courses for 15–30 days.

Typically, oral steroids will bring about a much greater decrease in the swelling in the nose and sinuses. In addition, it will control lower respiratory complaints such as inflammation related to asthma or bronchitis and will decrease any other inflammation in your body. Many of my patients who take steroids for their sinuses often comment that the steroids made their achy bones feel better as well.

How to take Oral Corticosteroids

Oral steroids are strong medicine but are very effective and safe when used properly. They are bitter to the taste, even in pill form. Be sure to eat something before taking this medication, and have a glass of water in hand when placing the tablets into your mouth. If there is nothing in your stomach, you might find that the steroids will upset it, which can cause gastroesophageal reflux.

Side Effects Steroids are excellent medicine with a bad reputation. Patient fears about taking steroids are usually way out of proportion to the risk of taking them. However, when using oral steroids at higher doses, the body's pituitary axis may shift, and you may experience weight gain, water retention, acne, irritability, breast enlargement, aggression, gastrointestinal upset, high blood pressure, palpitations, increased cholesterol levels, heart disease, impotence, liver failure, glaucoma, cataracts, and/or loss of sleep. Furthermore, steroids can make some people feel hungry and others feel bloated and have no appetite. Oddly, the loss of sleep caused by steroids is not related to insomnia: Even with fewer hours of sleep, these patients awake feeling alert and refreshed. These side effects rarely occur with short-term steroid usage.

Oral Steroids
Dexamethasone (Decadron)
Methylprednisolone (Medrol Dose pack)
Prednisolone (Pediapred, Orapred)
Prednisone (Deltasone, Orasone, Liquid Pred)

Topical Nasal Corticosteroids
Steroid nasal sprays deliver a precise dosage of medication directly to the nose and the sinuses and are far safer than oral steroids that have to travel through your body to take effect. Nasal steroid sprays have a very minimal uptake into the bloodstream, and this small amount gets excreted from the body fairly quickly. You must take your steroid nasal sprays every day for them to be effective, even when you are not suffering from symptoms. The steroid must work on your nasal membrane by bringing down membrane inflammation before it becomes effective; you may be using the spray anywhere from 3 days to 4 weeks before you will feel the benefits. The amount of time before feeling relief depends

on your dosage, your sensitivity to the medicines, your particular clinical picture, the specific steroid medication that is prescribed, and the way that your body reacts to it. Furthermore, if you are placed on additional oral steroids, then you will find that they augment any affect that topical steroids would have offered. Nasal steroid sprays have very few side effects and are safe to take. In addition, unlike over-the-counter decongestant sprays, there is no rebound phenomenon or any addiction.

Side Effects Nasal steroid sprays usually do not build up a systemic level because most of the steroid is minimally absorbed and that which gets absorbed gets eliminated by the body almost immediately. Because of this, most of the systemic effects of oral steroids are usually not experienced. The side effects even from a short-term, high-dose oral steroid are probably very low. The side effects of a nasal steroid spray are even lower. You will want to get regular checkups from your prescribing doctor if you will be using steroid nasal sprays for more than a few months, so that your progress, and any side effects, can be monitored.

The side effects of steroid nasal sprays include various sensations inside the nose (burning, dryness, or irritation), headaches, sore throat, or increased sneezing. These reactions are generally mild, and you should inform your physician if you are suffering from any of them. If you start to develop nosebleeds, stop using the spray immediately and consult your doctor. Steroid nasal sprays have been known to cause septal perforation (a hole in your septum between your two nostrils). This is probably caused by the propellant that carries the steroid rather than from the steroid itself or by the way that you insert the spray into your nose. Septal perforation from steroid sprays is a very rare complication.

Who Shouldn't Use Steroids

You should not use steroids of any type if you are pregnant (unless their use is approved by an obstetrician-gynecologist), you have glaucoma (unless approved by an ophthalmologist, or eye doctor), or you have diabetes (unless approved by an endocrinologist). Those with an allergy to the spray or who have had a previous untoward response should also not use it.

Nasal Corticosteroid Sprays

Beclomethasone (Beconase AQ)
Budesonide (Rhinocort Aqua)
Flunisolide (Nasarel, Nasalide)
Fluticasone (Flonase)

Mometasone (Nasonex)
Triamcinolone (Nasacort AQ)
Dexamethasone (Decadron
  Turbinaire)

Ophthalmic Corticosteroids

Ophthalmic steroids are used when the eye is inflamed from allergy and/or infection. These eye drops will reduce swelling and inflammation.

Fluromethalone (FML)
Loteprednol (Alrex)
Prednisolone (Pred Fate)

ANTIHISTAMINES

Histamines are chemicals the body releases during an allergic reaction. When an allergen is present, the body creates the histamine that binds itself to receptor cells in nasal tissues, nerve endings, and nearby blood vessels. These blood vessels begin to enlarge and leak fluid and increase mucus production, which leads to sneezing, itching, redness, and swelling. The end result is nasal congestion, wheezing, or irritated skin. Antihistamines prevent the histamine from binding to the histamine site by getting to these same places first: The antihistamine chemicals bind themselves to the receptor cells.

If you take antihistamines before exposure to an allergen, you may not develop symptoms. After the exposure has already taken place and some histamine has bound to the receptor cells, the antihistamine is not effective and will not reverse the allergic process. Instead, it stops the continuation of the allergic response going forward. That's why you will frequently see antihistamine medications combined with a decongestant medication. The antihistamine keeps further allergic reactions

The Josephson Technique for Applying Nasal Steroid Spray

These directions that follow are my personal recommendations for using nasal sprays. My directions differ from the directions in most package inserts for nasal steroid sprays. I recommend that you check with your physician before using my technique and before taking the medicine.

1. Shake the bottle.

2. Place the tip of the bottle into your right nostril, so that your fingers are up against your nostril. Hold the spray in your right hand for the right nostril.

3. Once inside the nostril, aim the tip toward the right eye.

4. Press the spray to allow one dose of the solution to go into your nose.

5. Do the same thing on the left side, aiming the nozzle toward the left eye. Use your left hand for administering the solution to the left nostril.

6. Breathe in and out slowly and deeply through your nose. This allows you to coat the membranes with the nasal spray by bringing the solution up and down coating the membranes of your nose.

7. Breathe slowly in and out through your nose with a closed mouth about 10 times.

8. Repeat steps 2–7 one more time.

from occurring, while the decongestant deals with symptoms already in the works. Antihistamines are found in both OTC and prescription formulations. They also appear in pill, liquid, nasal spray, and eyedrop forms.

Antihistamines will relieve only the symptoms related to allergies: If you are taking the medication correctly, the antihistamine will stop or quell the allergic symptom response. This will include nasal and sinus swelling, sneezing, itching, hives, and asthmatic flare.

Unfortunately, antihistamines are probably the most abused medicines available. Antihistamines will not work if you do not suffer from allergies, yet many physicians incorrectly prescribe antihistamines for their patients who have a cold even when the patient does not have allergies. Furthermore, patients very often self-prescribe OTC antihistamines or combination medicines that include antihistamines whether or not they have allergies.

For example, you might decide to take an antihistamine if you have a cold or for acute, recurrent acute or chronic sinusitis, believing that the antihistamine will dry up your congestion. But this is not the case. If allergies are not the cause of your sinus infection (and certainly they are never the cause of a cold) an antihistamine will do nothing. They will not disrupt the mucus production, clear the infection, or decrease nasal congestion. If you have congestion and mucus production with a sinus problem, a decongestant would be a better choice.

Who Shouldn't Use Antihistamines

Antihistamines are contraindicated for people with urinary tract obstruction, prostate enlargement, glaucoma, stomach ulcers, liver disease, intestinal obstruction, kidney disease, or a known allergy to the specific antihistamine.

Risks and Side Effects

Common side effects of antihistamines are sedation; dry mouth, nose, and eyes; excitation in children; and thickening of respiratory secretions. More severe side effects, when the medicine is used for a long period of time, include glaucoma, prostate enlargement, and stomach ulcers.

Combination Products

The main selling feature of combination medicines is that one pill (or liquid dose) will resolve many of your symptoms. These include "allergy and cold relief " and "sinus pain and headache" remedies. They are available over the counter as well as in prescription dosages. However, I recommend staying away from combinations unless you have discussed them with your doctor. Combination medicines often contain elements that you might not need, and you will bear the negative side effects of that element even though it is not doing anything for you. For example, a decongestant with a built-in antihistamine will make you more tired than you would feel by taking the decongestant alone. Furthermore, you risk experiencing the side effects of the antihistamine you do not need.

First-Generation Oral Antihistamines
Be sure to read the box your medicine comes in to determine its primary ingredients. Many products contain the following drugs in some combination with other agents.

> Brompheniramine, available as a combination product (Dimetapp)
> Chlorpheniramine (Chlor-Trimeton)
> Clemastine (Tavist)
> Cyproheptadine (Periactin, prescription only)
> Dexbrompheniramine, available as a combination product (Drixoral)
> Diphenhydramine (Benadryl)
> Promethazine (Phenergan, prescription only)

Second-Generation Oral Antihistamines
Products labeled "D" also contain the decongestant pseudoephedrine.

> Acrivastine (Semprex-D, prescription only)
> Cetirizine (Zyrtec, Zyrtec-D, prescription only)
> Desloratadine (Clarinex RediTabs, prescription only)
> Fexofenadine (Allegra, Allegra-D, prescription only)
> Loratadine (Claritin, Dimetapp ND, Alavert, Claritin RediTabs, Claritin-D)

Topical Nasal Antihistamines
Topical nasal antihistamines work in the same fashion as oral antihistamines and have minimal side effects. This type of nasal spray does not cause a rebound effect. It is usually prescribed for patients with sinus and/or nasal problems caused by allergy. One type is azelastine (Astelin), available by prescription only.

Topical Ophthalmic Antihistamines

Topical ophthalmic antihistamines are used when the eyes are severely affected by an allergic reaction. These eye drops will reduce swelling, itching, and tearing in and around the eye.

Azelastine (Optivar)

Emedastine (Emadine)

Levocabastine (Livostin)

Ketotifen (Zaditor)

Olopatadine (Patanol)

Antazoline/naphazoline, an antihistamine/decongestant combination (Vasocon-A)

Epinastine (Elestat)

Pheniramine/naphazoline, an antihistamine/decongestant combination (Naphcon-A, Visine-A)

DECONGESTANTS

During an allergic reaction or other inflammation, tissues in the nose and blood vessels in the eyes and other areas swell. At the same time, mucus builds up in the nasal cavity. All of these effects result in a runny and/or stuffy nose and red eyes. Decongestants work by constricting the blood vessels in your eyes and nose, shrinking swollen nasal tissues, and reducing blood flow to the mucous membranes.

Decongestants offer symptomatic relief of nasal congestion due to the common cold, allergies, or sinusitis. Decongestants may also aid in nasal or sinus drainage. These medications are generally available in many forms including pills, liquid or syrup, and nasal spray.

Who Shouldn't Use Oral Decongestants

People who take monoamine oxidase (MAO) inhibitors, have uncontrolled high blood pressure, heart disease, glaucoma, prostate enlargement, or allergy to these agents should avoid decongestants. Many physicians recommend decongestants as a long-term solution for chronic sinusitis. I do not recommend this class of medicines for more than 1 week because

I believe the long-term effects can be dangerous. Decongestants have stimulant-like properties. Often, you might find that while taking decongestants you have a temporary increase in alertness as well as relief from fatigue. This stimulating influence can have an effect on your heart and your sleep patterns and, in men, can affect the prostate. Any use for more than 72 hours should be under the supervision of a physician.

Risks and Side Effects
Some side effects of decongestants are increased blood pressure, increased heart rate, palpitations, nervousness, insomnia, dizziness, tremor, sweating, and rebound congestion with topical nasal agents. Topical decongestants should not be used for more than 2 days at a time to prevent rebound congestion.

Oral Decongestants
Just as with antihistamines, it's important to read the information on the medicine's box. Many products contain these two drugs in various combinations with other agents: pseudoephedrine (Sudafed) and phenylephrine (Sudafed PE).

Decongestant Nasal Sprays
OTC nasal sprays may be effective in the short term but will be very harmful in the long term. These popular products appear at first to be effective because they shrink the nasal tissues so that you can breathe more freely. However, after repeated use, the tissues become swollen and rebound. This rebound swelling is actually worse than the original swelling: The product eventually becomes ineffective and your sinus congestion worsens. This condition is called "rhinitis medicamentosa." In addition, these products can actually irreversibly damage the membranes of the nose and the sinuses. Septal perforation can occur secondary to decongestant nasal spray overuse.

Topical Nasal Decongestants
Naphazoline (Privine)
Oxymetazoline (Afrin)

Phenylephrine (Neo-Synephrine)
Tetrahydrozoline (Tyzine, prescription only)

TOPICAL NASAL ANTICHOLINERGIC AGENTS

Anticholinergic products offer temporary relief of runny nose. They work by decreasing nasal secretions and blocking receptor sites that cause mucus production. One anticholinergic agent is ipratropium (Atrovent). Patients who are allergic to the medication ipratropium should not take these products. Side effects include bloody nose, nasal dryness, and nausea.

MUCOLYTICS

Mucolytics cause the goblet cells to increase the amount of water in the mucus, which changes the consistency to be thinner and flow more easily. These medications are prescribed for people whose major symptoms are thickened mucus and postnasal drip. They act as expectorants, helping the body loosen mucus by making bronchial secretions thinner and easier to cough up; they do not suppress a cough. These agents are usually an adjunct medication within a broader remedy treatment protocol. One example is guaifenesin (Mucinex and Humibid plain).

NASAL EMOLLIENTS, ANTISEPTICS, AND GELS

Nasal emollients and gels allow mucus to glide over dry ciliated hair cells so that it can move through the sinuses with ease. These are useful for soothing your dry nasal membranes when you have a cold, suffer from allergies, fly a lot, are in a dry climate, are pregnant, or are using oxygen therapy. One very useful application for these preparations is to treat nosebleeds caused by dryness. They are also useful in preventing discomfort from having a dry, crusty nose.

New antiseptic products have recently come out as OTC medications (SinoFresh). They appear to kill bacteria and fungus. However, further testing needs to be performed to evaluate their effects on the nasal membranes and ciliated hair cells.

Some nasal emollients and gels are Ayr Nasal Gel, Borolcum, and Ponaris.

THROAT SPRAYS AND LOZENGES

Throat sprays are appropriate when you are experiencing a sore throat caused by postnasal drip or during an acute flare-up of a chronic infection. Some products may contain an antiseptic that kills bacteria and fungus as it passes into the throat. Other functions of these products include coating the throat, reducing the inflammation and the pain of a sore throat, and facilitating easier swallowing. Products that are available for sore throat relief contain topical anesthetics such as phenol (Chloraseptic), hexylresorcinols (Sucrets), benzocaine (Goldberger's Super Troche Plus), and methanol (Cepacol).

COUGH SUPPRESSANTS

Codeine and hydrocodone are prescription cough suppressants. Dextromethorphan is an oral cough suppressant that is available in many OTC cough and cold remedies. Dextromethorphan is chemically related to codeine and acts on the brain to suppress cough but does not have the pain-relieving and addictive properties of codeine.

ANTISEPTIC MOUTH WASHES

Mouth washes reduce the amount of bacteria in the mouth, teeth, and gums related to sinus infections that can cause gingivitis, dental infections, and halitosis (bad breath).

CHEST RUBS

Chest rubs are OTC medications formulated to be placed on the chest. They provide heat to the chest, which can help warm the lungs and reduce inflammation. Some people mistakenly place this medication in and around the nose to achieve similar results. This is not a good idea because proper studies of this use have not been performed and some researchers believe that these products may cause negative effects on the mucous membranes and ciliated hair cells.

ANTIFUNGAL TREATMENT

Fungus and mold are always present in the air, so it is reasonable to expect that they are also found in our nasal passages. Recent research at the Mayo Clinic has confirmed this to be true. In people with CAID, an immune response to the fungi results in a thickening of the mucous membrane, leading to the disease's symptoms. The presence of fungus triggers certain white blood cells to secrete substances that attract other white blood cells to defend the body against the fungus, which in normal patients may be harmless. These white blood cells secrete a protein called major basic protein (MBP), a substance that is directly toxic to the fungi. However, MBP can also damage the sensitive nasal mucous membrane. Over time, this damage leads to swelling and breaks in the membrane. It can also make the mucous membrane vulnerable to invasion by other bacterial and viral organisms.

Clinical studies at the Mayo Clinic have demonstrated that topical antifungals are effective in treating and altering the disease progression of CAID by eliminating fungal elements that can exacerbate the disease. In addition, studies of topical antifungal therapies have demonstrated that the agents can decrease mucous membrane swelling and thickening.

CAID patients who use topical antifungal drugs avoid the side effects common with oral and intravenous antifungal formulations. Topical administration allows a high dose to be applied to the fungus while limiting the patient's exposure to the drug. Side effects reported by patients are minimal but include burning and worsening of congestion.

In clinical studies, the following topical antifungals have been used at the indicated doses:

Amphotericin B: 100 mg/L of sterile water (up to 200 mg/L has been used)

Itraconazole: 100–200 mg/L of sterile water

Voriconazole: 1000 mg/L of normal saline

ANTIVIRAL PREVENTATIVE MEASURES

It has been shown that yearly flu shots are effective in decreasing the incidence of flu in patients. Typically, people with the flu will experience sinusitis symptoms, which can be prevented with the vaccine.

Sinus Friendly Foods

In the 12th century, the physician Moses Maimonides first prescribed chicken soup as a cold and asthma remedy. People have experienced the same tried-and-true results over the centuries, but the true therapeutic properties of chicken soup, however, have not been studied until recently. Just as your grandmother may have told you, chicken soup does help relieve the symptoms of colds and flu. Good news for vegetarians: The vegetables in the soup have some of the same qualities as the chicken.

Dr. Stephen Rennard, a chest specialist at the University of Nebraska Medical Center in Omaha, tested various chicken soups, from a traditional, home-made soup to a number of commercial varieties. Rennard found that chicken soup had anti-inflammatory properties that acted to stop sore throats. He found that the soup helped stop the movement of neutrophils (white blood cells that encourage the flow of mucus). As a result, chicken soup has been found to relieve patients who suffer from the flu. Irwin Ziment, M.D., a pulmonary specialist and professor at the University of California at Los Angeles's School for Medicine, found that chicken soup contains drug-like agents similar to those in modern cold medicines. For example, an amino acid released from chicken during cooking chemically resembles the drug acetylcysteine, prescribed for bronchitis and other respiratory problems. Spices that are often added to chicken soup, such as garlic and

Grandma Josephson's Homemade Chicken Soup

SERVES 4 TO 6

One 3–4 lb. pullet chicken
1 1 lb. package of chicken
  wings and giblets
1 large tomato, cut in half
3 large yellow onions, quartered
3 parsnips, quartered

2 turnips, quartered
11–12 large carrots, sliced
1 bunch fresh parsley
5–6 celery ribs
1 bunch fresh dill
Salt and pepper to taste

Clean the chicken. Put the chicken in a large pot and cover it with cold water. Bring the water to a boil. Add the wings, giblets, tomato, onions, parsnips, turnips, and carrots. Simmer about 1 1/2 hours. Remove the fat from the surface of the broth as it accumulates. Add the parsley, dill, and celery. Cook the soup about 45 minutes longer. Remove the chicken. Put the vegetables in a food processor and process until they are chopped fine, or pass through a strainer. Add salt and pepper to taste.

pepper (all ancient treatments for respiratory diseases), work the same way as modern cough medicines, thinning mucus and making breathing easier.

Other researchers believe that it is not the soup but the steam it gives off that holds the real benefit. Sipping hot soup and breathing in the steam helps clear up congestion. Others say that hot water is not as helpful as chicken soup, although it may be soothing to our throats, especially if you add honey and lemon.

Supplements and Nutrients

A balanced diet high in protein, fruits, and vegetables is very important for patients suffering from CAID. For patients who get frequent infections, I recommend supplementing their diet with a multivitamin as well as a high dose of vitamins B and C.

Moving to Another State

In the past, physicians recommended that their patients with chronic sinusitis and/or allergies move to another part of the country, where the climate was different, thinking that they could either avoid the allergies in that area or avoid a climate that causes them to have problems. Usually, a warmer, dryer climate was recommended. However, most of these people found that the move would help their symptoms only for a very short time. In actuality, your sinuses will catch up with the pollutants or irritants in the new community, and very shortly you may be suffering from the local climate. What's more, many people brought with them infectious agents and plants from their original location, so the pollens from the plants where they used to live were still around, but in smaller quantities. So unless you are planning to move to the moon or to an area where there are no other inhabitants, this solution will not be permanent.

CHAPTER 5

CONTROLLING ALLERGIES, FOOD SENSITIVITIES, AND AIRBORNE IRRITANTS

Allergy symptoms can easily be mistaken for the common cold in much the same way as the other signs and symptoms of chronic airway-digestive inflammatory disease (CAID). In fact, the allergic response is actually one of the main causes leading to CAID: Allergies left untreated will cause inflammation to the sinus membranes, spawning the cascade of swelling and obstruction. Once this occurs, you may experience the same congestion, headaches, postnasal drip, hoarseness, and so on that you would feel during a bout of sinusitis. On top of these symptoms, you may also experience certain symptoms that pertain to the allergic reaction, including:

- Asthma
- Eczema
- Food allergy
- Hives
- Itchy, watery eyes
- Runny nose
- Sneezing

Allergies can seriously affect your quality of life. Allergies will persist for as long as you are exposed to the allergen. If you have environmental allergies, such as pollen or ragweed, your symptoms can last as long as a few weeks to more than a few months. Severe allergies require more than a standard cold medication. Untreated allergy symptoms can also develop into more chronic conditions, such as ear infections and sinusitis.

Doctors are still unclear as to why some patients with allergies develop sinus disease, nasal polyps, and asthma, while other's allergic reactivity manifests itself in rashes and/or itching. I believe that each individual's genetic map must code for the areas to be affected (known as target areas) by the inflammatory process that erupts with an allergic reaction.

Because the allergic response and the symptoms of sinus disease and CAID are so similar, it is often difficult for anyone, including a doctor, to differentiate between the two.

My patient Steven came to the office complaining of continuous nasal congestion, postnasal drip, and headaches. He told me that he felt as if he were always suffering from some kind of sinus-related symptom. His problems start in the beginning of the spring each year and last through the fall. He sneezes at times and has itchy eyes in the fall when it is windy. Steven complained that his mucus usually turns yellow in the fall when the weather gets colder, although he claimed that it is clear and white throughout the spring and summer. Once the winter starts, his symptoms improve dramatically, except for an occasional 2- to 3-day cold. He started self-medicating with over-the-counter (OTC) remedies, including decongestant nasal sprays. He was also being treated by a health-food store with various vitamins and holistic products. These supplements do make him feel better but not good enough: He said that he used his nasal spray every 2–3 hours. Worse, Steven couldn't sleep because he couldn't breathe through his nose at night, and his wife said he had begun to snore.

Steven went to an allergist who said that he did not have allergies and treated him with an antibiotic for 7 days and a nasal spray for 2 weeks. However, Steven was never tested for allergies, and his symptoms didn't improve. Another ear, nose, and throat (ENT) specialist did a computed tomography (CT) scan and recommended surgery. Steven's internist recommended various antihistamines and decongestants and kept putting him on a 5-day course of antibiotics, which offered some improvement but never seemed to do the trick.

Steven came to my office, and I took a history and performed a physical examination. I sat down and spoke with Steven and let him know that I thought he suffered from allergic rhinitis, which turned into a chronic sinusitis in the fall. During the examination I listened to his chest and heard a slight wheezing. He told me that this often happened in the spring or fall, but it never bothered him enough to treat. His biggest pressing problem was the rhinitis medicamentosa that he developed from the topical decongestant. He was addicted to his nasal spray, was rebounding from the medicine, and was worse than ever. I recommended that he see another allergist for allergy testing. I sent him to an osteopath for control of his supplements and his holistic medicines. I placed him on a course of nasal steroid sprays and oral steroids and decongestants for 2 weeks and told him in no uncertain terms to quit taking the topical decongestant spray immediately.

Steven came back to my office 2 weeks later. He told me that he went cold turkey on the decongestant spray, even though the first 2 nights were extremely tough. By the end of the 1st week, he no longer thought about using the decongestant spray. His snoring stopped as his breathing retuned to near normal. I then put him on an antibiotic for 30 days, which cleared up his yellow discharge. He reported that his allergy testing was positive, and the allergist instituted an allergy-shot protocol. We placed him on a nasal steroid spray and an antihistamine over the next year.

By the next spring Steven told me that he was barely feeling his old allergy symptoms. He breezed through to the next spring without an infection. He stated he wheezed maybe once a year when the pollen got really bad but even then it was barely noticeable. On his own, Steven learned how to use a nasal irrigator when the allergy season is in full swing. Overall, Steven feels like a new man.

The Allergic Reaction

A person becomes allergic when he or she acquires an abnormal immune response to a substance that does not normally cause a reaction. This typically occurs after an initial exposure (sensitization) to the allergen, although multiple exposures to the substance may be necessary.

There is apparently a genetic predisposition to allergies; the incidence is higher in children whose parents also suffer. If one parent is allergic, the incidence is roughly 29 percent and if both parents are allergic the likelihood that the child will have allergies increases to about 47 percent. However, allergies can develop during any stage in life: You are not simply born "allergic." There is an allergic continuum on which during the course of your life there are times where you are more likely to become allergic than others. Some patients outgrow their allergy, which means that they are no longer affected. Years later, the same allergy might reappear. What's more, allergies can affect different target organs at different times. This may be the case as the sensitivity of the target organ may change over time. For example, you may suffer from a different pattern of allergy symptoms today than you did 10 years ago, and it may change in the future.

The allergen must enter a person's body for it to trigger an immune response. This can happen through physical contact (something on the hand that gets transferred to the eyes, nose, mouth, or ears), inhalation, ingestion, or injection (drugs). The next time the exposure occurs, a broad spectrum of inflammatory responses will begin, causing an allergic reaction. What's happening to your body is this: The immune system that is responsible for protecting the body from harmful foreign substances is presented with a substance that it cannot tolerate. For example, when the immune system is confronted with an allergen such as pollen, it mistakes it for a foreign, invasive substance, even though pollen is not typically harmful to most people. Yet the allergic reaction may be devastating to the point at which it can make the allergic person very sick and can even be deadly.

The typical immune response to any foreign substance—be it a virus, bacteria, cancer cell, or allergen—is to form an antibody or im-munoglobulin to that antigen. For instance, when you contract a strept infection of the nose or throat, a whole series of reactions occur that defend you from that bacteria. Antibodies are formed to the *Streptococ-cus* bacteria. They attach to the *Streptococcus pneumoniae* cell membrane and attack the bacteria directly, while also instructing your white blood cells to attack, engulf and kill the bacteria.

In the case of an allergy, your body perceives the pollen as a threat. You start to form an antibody against pollen. This antibody is called im-munoglobulin E (IgE). The IgE binds to white blood cells called mast cells and basophils. Mast cells are found in connective tissue all over the body, especially located near small blood vessels. Basophils are found in the bloodstream. When there is an allergic reaction, these cells migrate toward the nasal membrane. Mast cells and basophils contain histamine and other chemical mediators of inflammation that they release like little explosives. So when pollen enters your body, it comes into contact with the IgE bound to a mast cell or the basophil. The mast cell or basophil explodes, releasing histamine and other inflammatory substances, which cause swelling, heat, and often itching: the allergic response.

There are two phases to the allergic response. The first is an early response, which occurs within seconds of the introduction of the anti-gen. This immediate response lasts for only a few minutes. The second response occurs when the white blood cells are launched during the in-flammatory response. However, symptoms can occur during either the early or the late reaction.

Antigen exposure will lead to itching within seconds, followed by sneezing. A runny nose follows, and within about 15 minutes you will become congested and stuffy. You may also complain about tearing, itchy eyes, sore throat, throat clearing and coughing, itchy throat and ears, and ear popping. Sinus obstruction due to the swelling and con-gestion can lead to sinusitis, when the connection with CAID begins. Nasal obstruction leads to mouth breathing, snoring, and sleep apnea. Eustachian tube dysfunction may occur, leading to hearing loss, tinnitus (ringing in the ear), and/or dizziness (vertigo). The gastrointestinal tract can then be affected as the infected mucus travels into the stomach, and you may complain of any of the following symptoms: gas, belching, bloating, indigestion, diarrhea, and ingestional fatigue (a feeling of tiredness following a meal).

In children this can lead to adenoid infections and abnormal dental development. In addition, these children usually have "allergic shiners," dark circles around the eyes, and swollen eye lids. Children can also develop a horizontal crease along the tip of their nose from rubbing it so often (affectionately called "the allergic salute").

Decoding My Problem

Review your results from the allergy portion of the CAID Quiz (p. 71). Locate your score so you can define your next course of action. Follow these guidelines:

The Difference between Rhinitis and Allergic Rhinitis

As you've learned, *rhinitis* refers to inflammation and swelling of the nose. Rhinitis can be allergic or nonallergic. Hay fever and rose fever are two common terms that we use to describe allergic rhinitis. Both terms are misnomers in that hay fever is not a reaction to (or fever caused by) hay. And rose fever is not an allergy to roses (despite what most people think, there are no allergies to flowers). Symptoms of allergic rhinitis can begin at any age but are most frequently reported in adolescence and young adulthood. Allergic rhinitis is caused by an allergen, whereas nonallergic rhinitis is caused by a different set of components, including hot spicy food, environmental irritants like strong odors, cigarette smoke, car exhaust, chemicals, sudden changes in temperature and humidity and cold air exposure. However, it's possible to experience allergic and nonallergic rhinitis at the same time. This can make it very difficult for your physician to diagnose. My patient Steven suffered from both allergic rhinitis and nonallergic rhinitis, the latter being caused by the decongestant spray.

- If your score is 0–10 then you can treat yourself with OTC medicines
- If your score is 11–25 then you need to see your primary-care physician
- If your score is 26–45 then you need to see an allergist or an otolaryngologic allergist
- If your score is 46 or more then you need to see an ENT who specializes in treating CAID or at least specializes in allergies

If you frequently sneeze, have a runny nose, congestion, and itchy eyes all year long then you suffer from perennial allergies that include pollution, animals, or dust. These recurrent allergies may be more subtle, making it harder for you and/or your physician to diagnose.

If you suffer from these symptoms only in the spring, summer, or fall, it is more likely that you suffer from seasonal allergies connected to different plant or mold growths. Tree pollen falls when the trees begin to bloom in the early spring. Grass pollens are the culprit starting in the late spring or early summer. By late July, your allergies will calm down as tree and grass pollen counts typically drop. The end of the summer or the early part of fall will bring in ragweed pollen season. These pollens remain a nuisance until the early winter with the first frost. The freezing temperature will kill the weed plants, and your allergies will take a breather until the following year. Those of you who think you are insulated from allergies in the big cities, because there are not many trees, think again. Grass, tree, and weed pollens are small particles that are carried for miles by the wind. Some sufferers will tell you that their allergies are worse in the city, because they are not only inundated with pollens but are also hit with nonallergic rhinitis from the car exhaust and other pollution.

Many with allergies have mild symptoms. These people may choose to live with them or medicate themselves with OTC allergy medicines. Then there are the patients who are miserable as a result of their allergies. Some are even debilitated. Lastly, although rare, allergic reactions, such as bee stings or food allergies, can be deadly. For anyone whose allergies are more than an annoyance, I strongly advise seeking professional help as soon as possible.

Choosing an Allergist

Allergists receive their accreditation in two distinct ways: either by the American Academy of Allergy or by the American Academy of Otolaryngology. Both are equally well trained and proficient in treating allergies.

Your Appointment with an Allergist

Just like your appointment with your primary-care physician or any other specialist, your visit with an allergist begins by taking your medical history and conducting a thorough physical examination. The doctor should be checking for allergic reactions involving the skin, eyes, ears, nose, throat, and neck but should also examine areas affected by CAID, including your chest, heart, lungs, abdomen, and general nervous system.

Your physician should also ask you the following:

- What is the chief (main) complaint that has brought you to the office?
- What are the symptoms that accompany your chief complaint? How long do they last? When do they occur? When did the symptom first appear? What medicines do you take and for what problem are you taking them?
- Have you had previous surgery? What type and when?
- Do you have any allergies to medicines that you know about? What type of reaction did you get?
- Do you have any seasonal or all-year-round allergies that you know about?

Next, your doctor should ask you questions regarding every system in your body: head, neck, nose, mouth, ears, eyes, chest, heart, lungs, legs, arms, back, and so on. This is called a review of systems.

> ## Check Your Pollen Count
>
> The Internet is a great resource for checking pollen counts. Often, a local radio station provides this information on its website. You can also check national websites, if you will be traveling.

ALLERGY TESTING

The next part of the exam will involve allergy testing to determine what allergies you may have, including ones you may not be aware of. This testing can be performed via various methods. An allergist typically uses the scratch or prick test as a primary tool for allergy testing. The intradermal skin endpoint titration test is believed by some to be more accurate. And more recently, technology has brought about blood testing called the radioallergosorbent test (RAST). Each of these tests has their strengths and weaknesses, and you should speak with your physician to decide which he or she feels is best for you.

Occasionally, a person is acutely aware of his or her allergies, but the testing is negative. This result is called a false negative. Most physicians will choose to continue to treat with allergy medicine, using the medication itself as a test. You may be asked to take the prescribed antihistamine for a time, then stop, and start again if symptoms get worse after stopping. If the antihistamine provides relief, then there is a good chance that you suffer from allergies even though your test was negative.

ADDITIONAL BLOOD TESTING

Your allergist may want to see a detailed report of your blood. He or she may send it to the laboratory to see if you have high levels of IgE. Furthermore, he or she may also want to evaluate your immunoglobulin G (IgG) levels if you have bad sinus disease, although these tests are not commonly performed. Your physician will usually do this only if he or she feels that there is an immunologic problem leading to recurrent sinus infections.

NASAL TESTING

Your physician may want to do a nasal smear. He or she will collect some of your nasal mucus and then look at it under a microscope. Your physician will be looking for white blood cells in the mucus. If he or she identifies eosinophils and goblet cells in your mucus then you suffer from pollen and/or inhalant allergies. If he or she finds basophils then you may have a food allergy. Neutrophils indicate an inflammatory reaction and this white cell can be found with allergy or infection.

Primary Allergy Treatment: Avoidance

Just like there is no cure for CAID, there is no cure for allergies. However, with new techniques and medications, it is possible to live without experiencing the troubling symptoms associated with them.

The most direct way to limit your allergic symptoms is through a few lifestyle changes, most notably by avoiding the known allergen entirely. This is easier said than done. Luckily, there are many new tools and techniques to make avoidance a practical part of your life.

PERENNIAL ALLERGENS

Because you feel sick all year long, it's really important to eliminate the particular allergen from your surroundings. The most common perennial allergens are house dust mites, animal dander from your pets, feathers from pillows and comforters, and cockroaches.

Household dust is found all over the world. It is actually a combination of allergens. It is different from road dust in that road dust is an irritant; although at certain times of the year, like autumn, road dust can contain allergic mold spores. Household dust is a combination of breakdown products from your carpets and upholstery, including down and lint products, debris including human skin flakes and animal dander, plant matter, cockroach fragments, bacteria, and mold. Household dust also provides a home for dust mites. There are over 50,000 species of these microscopic insects that feed on your skin as it sheds. These bugs tend to accumulate in mattresses, pillows, carpeting, and upholstered furniture. Oriental rugs, English tweed fabrics, down pillows and comforters create thriving environments for dust mites. They also prefer more humid environments so that homes in higher altitudes like Denver or the western desert states have less problems than homes in more humid states like New York or sunny, tropical Florida.

Reactions to household dust are typically worse in the morning after a night's sleep, lying in the dust-mite-infested bedding. Vacuuming and shaking out bedding and/or rugs can trigger symptoms.

Avoidance and reducing exposure is the best way to help avoid these allergic reactions. Luckily, dust mites do not like plastic. The following are the steps that you need to take to minimize contact with these allergens:

1. Wash bedding weekly in hot water and dry in a hot dryer.
2. Remove carpeting, especially in the bedroom, and replace with hardwood or tile floors. You can keep area rugs or relatively new synthetic carpeting (less than 10 years old) if they are vacuumed weekly and washed or cleaned regularly. Chemical treatments with benzyl benzoate and other carpet and upholstery cleaners that are commercially available can be used to kill dust mites.
3. Place plastic covers on mattresses (box spring and mattress), pillows, and comforters to suffocate existing mites and keep new ones from hatching. Dust mites are usually not a problem in baby cribs as the mattresses are usually plastic covered.
4. Use dehumidifiers to lower the humidity, and run the air-conditioner in the summer to dry out your home.
5. Keep the carpeting dry. Do not walk on carpeting with wet feet or place wet towels on the carpeting or the bedding after showering. Take your shoes off at the front door so that you do not track in dust from your office or other people's homes.
6. Vacuum your entire home weekly. Make sure that your vacuum has a high-efficiency particulate air (HEPA) filter, which filters dirt particles in the air during vacuuming. The person in your home who is allergic should not do the vacuuming.

7. Wash down the walls, shelves, and floors regularly. Use single wipe dust rags and damp mops to clean around all surfaces. Or wash all cleaning rags in hot water after each use.

8. The best type of furniture to purchase is sealed wood, plastic, or metal with a minimum of stuffing. Keep heavy drapes to a minimum and keep Venetian blinds clean, as these surfaces are wonderful homes for the allergens.

HOUSEHOLD PETS

Allergies to your pets is a heartbreaking problem. I grew up with allergies to animals and I wanted to be a veterinarian. We had a dog, cats, and gerbils, and I loved horses. Allergies to indoor pets may not develop until months or even years after the first exposure. And by then these pets are family members. So if you are wondering if you have to get rid of your pets, my answer is always no. Try modification first.

Because you've been living with a pet or a house full of dust for a long time, the allergic reaction becomes chronic, ongoing, and continuous. Therefore you may not feel better even when you leave your house for the day. It may not be until you go on vacation for longer periods of time (more than 2 weeks) that you realize there is a problem. Or, upon returning, your symptoms begin again the moment you enter your home.

Most people think that they are allergic to the animal's fur. Actually, what you are allergic to is its dander, the protein from its skin that flakes off like dandruff on human scalps. Cat dander is lighter than dust mites and is carried in the air for long periods of time. It can also attach to the clothes of people who have cats, who then carry this dander out of the home and into work or school. This dander hangs around long after people no longer have a cat. Recent studies suggest that as the exposure to cat allergen increases, you can develop immunity to it, and it will no longer affect you.

Dog dander is also lightweight, but not as lightweight as cat dander. It has been shown that all breeds of cats usually cause a similar reaction, but in dogs, people can be sensitive to one breed but may not be sensitive to others. Some dogs also have hair instead of fur. Usually, dogs with hair can be tolerated, whereas dogs with fur cannot.

Horses (and their manure), gerbils, hamsters, mice, rats, rabbits, guinea pigs, and other furry rodents are also sources of allergen. Urine is the source of allergen for small animals, so the cage should not be kept in the room of the sufferer. Our feathered friends are messy in that they molt, preen themselves and shake feather debris all over the place. The feathers and the dust are sources of the allergic response.

While you might not want to get rid of these pets, reducing exposure to them is the best way to help avoid these allergic reactions. Follow the same guidelines listed for perennial allergens, and add these steps to protect you from your pets:

1. Restrict the range of your pets. Keep them out of the bedroom and any other room where you may spend a lot of time.
2. Carpeting in rooms where your pet lives should be vacuumed weekly and cleaned regularly. Hardwood, linoleum, or tile floors are better choices for pets, anyway.
3. Your pet should have a bed of its own, which should be located away from the allergic person. Dog and cat cases and cages must be kept clean. Cat litter boxes should be cleaned regularly and should not be changed by the allergic person.
4. Keep your pets clean and well groomed. Your pet should be washed at least once a week. All the towels that are used for drying must be immediately washed in hot water and dried. The allergic person should not be the person who brushes the pet.
5. Weather permitting, you may want to keep the pet outdoors or on a porch. This works only if you never let the animal in the house, because if it makes daily visits, then the dander will be in the house anyway.
6. After playing with a cat, dog, or furry friend or riding a horse (or gardening with horse manure), take a shower to wash the dander

from your skin and hair. Make sure that you do this before going into your bedroom. Change and wash your clothes immediately and do not bring your clothes into your bedroom. Certainly do not lie on your bed with this clothing before taking a shower, otherwise you will have transported the dander to your bedding and then you will sleep in it.

Unfortunately, if those suggestions do not help or if the allergy triggers significant asthma, it may be necessary to find your pet a new home. Remember, that if you give up your pet, it still takes a very long time for the allergen levels in your home to drop. It can take months. Aggressive cleaning such as removing the carpet, cleaning draperies, and washing the walls will hasten the process.

COCKROACHES

Cockroaches are a potent source of allergen. The cockroach allergen comes from the body parts of the cockroach and not the feces, as is the case with dust mites. Cockroach allergen was first found after many patients in the inner city came to public hospital emergency rooms with asthmatic flare-ups. They were found to have positive allergy tests to cockroach. On the other hand, positive tests for cockroach are rare in the suburbs.

Avoidance and reducing exposure to cockroaches is the best way to help avoid these allergic reactions. Cleaning of all areas around food and garbage and enclosure of all food and waste is important to keep away the cockroaches. Special glues and bait may be useful to get rid of cockroaches. There are many commercially available chemicals to kill these insects. Unfortunately, cockroach antigen may remain in homes for years after the last cockroach is gone.

SEASONAL ALLERGENS

Avoidance and reducing exposure is the best way to help avoid seasonal allergic reactions, especially when pollen counts are high. These are the steps that you need to take to minimize contact with these allergens:

1. Stay indoors, especially on high-pollen-count and windy days. Pollen counts are usually the highest in the morning so stay in during the morning hours.
2. Keep the windows and doors in your home closed to keep pollen out.
3. Turn on your air-conditioning units. Keep the vents closed and recirculate the air to remove the small amount of pollen that is in the air that has entered the house. Keep your air-conditioning filter clean and change it when it is dirty.
4. Use room air purifiers and filters. Keep them clean and be sure to change their filters. This will further eliminate pollens in the air in your home.
5. When in the car, keep the air-conditioning on in the recirculate position and keep the windows closed.
6. Do not go near cut grass and/or do not cut the lawn, as this will put pollen allergens into the air. For very allergic people, playing golf near cut grass may not be the best idea. Many people complain that their CAID is worse after they play golf.
7. Do not rake leaves because this will put mold allergen into the air, causing your allergies to flare if you are allergic to mold.
8. Do not use clotheslines to hang drying clothes outside as pollens will collect on them. If you do this with your sheets, you then will place them on your bed and lie in a bed of pollen.
9. Take your clothes off and wash them immediately when arriving at home as there will be pollen on your clothes. Shower before going to bed so that you wash off any pollen that might make your allergies flare at night.

NASAL IRRIGATION

Irrigation of your nose and sinuses using a neti pot or a nasal irrigator with sterile saline or other solutions will help wash out your nose and sinuses from the very particles that are causing your allergies. Follow the instructions in Chapter 4 on using a neti pot or nasal irrigator. This practice is especially important if you have seasonal allergies and have spent a large part of your day outdoors.

Medical Treatment for Allergies

In addition to avoidance, allergies can be successfully treated with medication. This may include a combination of antihistamines, decongestants, antihistamine nasal sprays and eye drops, nasal steroid sprays, anticholinergic sprays, and leukotrienes. I typically start my allergy patients with an inhaled nasal corticosteroid, an oral second-generation antihistamine, or both.

If you suffer from seasonal allergies, you need to begin medical therapy before the anticipated appearance of allergens and continue during the time of likely exposure. For example, if you are allergic to tree pollen and grasses, this would mean starting your medication before the appearance of tree pollen in the spring and continuing through the peak of the grass-pollen season in May and June.

ANTIHISTAMINES

Antihistamines do not destroy released histamine, nor do they interfere with histamine already bound to the receptor site. Instead, they block the receptor site and subsequently block the histamine from binding to the receptor.

Antihistamines fall into various categories. The first antihistamines that we developed were strongly sedating. These are called first-generation. Second-generation antihistamines were developed later, and are nonsedating.

Oral antihistamines are absorbed into the bloodstream and usually start to work within 60 minutes. They are most effective in the treatment of the following symptoms of allergic rhinitis: sneezing, nasal and ocular itching, and runny nose. Antihistamines have little or no effect on nasal congestion. That is why they are often prescribed in combination with a decongestant. However, although I believe that long-term use of antihistamines is advised when indicated, I believe that long-term use of decongestants should not be recommended because of their stimulant properties.

Side Effects
Side effects of antihistamines include sedation; dryness in the mouth, eyes, and throughout the body; gastrointestinal distress, cardiac arrhythmias, and prostatic hypertrophy.

Common Antihistamines
Cetirizine (Zyrtec)

Chlorpheniramine
  (Chlor-Trimeton)

Desloratadine (Clarinex)

Diphenhydramine (Benaedryl)

Fexofenadine (Allegra)

Loratadine (Claritin, Alavert)

ANTIHISTAMINE SPRAYS

Nasal antihistamines are considered to be similar in efficacy to oral antihistamines. Nosebleeds are a very rare side effect; a bitter taste can occur, and this can be minimized by tilting your head down. It can, but rarely does, cause, nausea. One type is azelastine (Astelin Nasal Spray).

DECONGESTANTS

Oral decongestants cause the blood vessels in the nose to constrict, and the mucous membranes and the turbinates to shrink. This essentially relieves nasal congestion, improving nasal air flow. The combination of a decongestant and an antihistamine is significantly more effective in reducing total nasal symptoms, including nasal congestion, than either agent is alone. However, I am opposed to using decongestants on a chronic basis because of the side effects.

Side Effects

Decongestants are stimulants; and if used too frequently, they can cause insomnia, nervousness, tremor, and palpitations with arrhythmias. Decongestants should be used cautiously for those with coronary artery disease, hypertension, diabetes, or hyperthyroidism and in those receiving monoamine oxidase inhibitors. The drug may also aggravate narrow-angle glaucoma and symptoms of bladder-neck obstruction. Two common decongestants are pseudoephedrine (Sudafed) and phenylephrine (Sudafed PE).

MAST CELL STABILIZER SPRAYS

Mast cell stabilizers have an anti-inflammatory effect because they inhibit the release of histamine, reducing the amount of histamines and other inflammatory substances released by the mast cells. These sprays must be administered every 4 hours, with the first dose given before the allergic reaction happens.

Side Effects

A bitter taste can occur, although this can be minimized by tilting your head down after spraying. It can, but rarely does, cause nausea and/or nose bleeds. One type is cromolyn (Nasalcrom Nasal Spray), an OTC product.

NASAL STEROID SPRAYS

Nasal steroids reduce multiple aspects of the inflammatory response and are the preferred treatment for mild allergic rhinitis. They have also been shown to decrease the response to allergens if used before an allergenic exposure. Clinically, it has been shown that nasal corticosteroids are more effective than antihistamines for nasal congestion and sneezing. Yet there is no significant difference between nasal corticosteroids and antihistamines in relieving eye itching and tearing symptoms.

The sprays take effect in about 1 week and reach maximum effectiveness in about 1 month.

Side Effects

The most common side effect of the sprays is nasal bleeding. Septal crusting and perforation (a small hole in the septum) can occur, although this is rare. I find that if you aim the spray away from the septum, this crusting is less likely to occur.

Nasal Corticosteroid Sprays

Beclomethasone (Beconase AQ)   Flunisolide (Nasarel, Nasalide)

Budesonide (Rhinocort Aqua)   Fluticasone (Flonase)

Dexamethasone (Decadron   Mometasone (Nasonex)
   Turbinaire)   Triamcinolone (Nasacort AQ)

TOPICAL AGENTS FOR OCULAR USE

A mast-cell stabilizer inhibits histamine release, and relieves allergic conjunctivitis (redness and itching). Three types are cromolyn (Crolom), nedocromil (Alocril), and lodoxamide (Alomide).

Antihistamine eye drops block histamine receptors and relieve allergic conjunctivitis. Two agents are ketorolac (Acular) and azelastine (Optivar).

LEUKOTRIENE BLOCKERS

Leukotriene blockers reduce mucosal inflammation. It is thought to be as effective as a second-generation antihistamine for the treatment of allergic rhinitis. However, the drug is not effective when used on its own. Instead, I use leukotriene blockers as an additional treatment for patients who do not have an adequate response to an antihistamine, a nasal corticosteroid, or both. This drug is also approved for asthma and can be helpful in patients with nasal polyps and/or aspirin allergy. The side effects are liver toxicity. One type is montelukast (Singulair).

ANTICHOLINERGIC AGENTS

Anticholinergic agents are effective for resolving a runny nose. It is approved, at one strength, for the common cold and is the drug of choice for such conditions as runny nose related to cold weather (skier's nose) and/or runny nose related to eating or just excessive postnasal drip. The side effects include headache and nosebleed, but these are very rare. One agent is ipratropium (Atrovent).

SYSTEMIC STEROIDS

Systemic steroids are usually reserved for severe symptoms that do not respond to other medications or for patients who cannot tolerate other drugs. In these cases, your physician may treat you with either oral or injected systemic corticosteroids. Treatment regimens include either a preseasonal intramuscular injection or oral corticosteroids, administered for a week to several weeks. For patients with severe allergies and asthma, long-term steroids may be necessary.

Side Effects

Systemic corticosteroid effects include adrenal suppression if used for more than 2 weeks. A short-term course of steroids may cause mood swings (especially for children) and increased hunger. Even a short-term course can lead to a lowering of the body's resistance to chickenpox, if you have not been exposed to this disease. Contact your doctor if you or your child are taking (or have just finished) oral steroids and come into contact with chickenpox. If your doctor thinks you are at risk he or she can give you an injection to protect you.

Long-term steroid administration (months or years) can have serious side effects. For these reasons your doctor should always try to prescribe the smallest possible dose. It is important that you continue all other treatments and take them regularly to keep the need for oral steroids to a minimum. The side effects of long-term oral steroid use include flattened face (moon face), feeling hungry and wanting to eat more (leading to weight gain), water retention, feeling hyped up and overactive, difficulty sleeping (although patients report that they don't feel tired), feeling depressed or experiencing sudden mood swings, heartburn and indigestion, bruising easily, brittle bones (osteoporosis), altering diabetic control or uncovering a tendency to diabetes, increased risk of cataract, and worsening of glaucoma.

Taking your steroids in the morning may decrease any side effects. Weight-bearing exercise, such as walking for 20 minutes each day will help protect against the bone thinning effect of long-term steroid use. Hormone-replacement therapy (HRT) in postmenopausal women reduces the risk of bone thinning and is advised in postmenopausal woman on long-term steroids. Continue taking topical nasal steroid sprays as this may decrease the need in dose or time for you to take oral steroids.

When you are taking oral steroids your adrenal gland becomes lazy and makes less of its own natural steroids. This means you have less ability to cope with infections or deal with physical stress. Long courses of steroids (3 weeks or more) can be stopped only by gradual reduction and under the guidance of a doctor. If they are stopped suddenly, you will be very vulnerable to infection and less able to cope with any crisis, such as an operation. For this reason, the doses should be reduced slowly over weeks or months.

Two oral agents are prednisone (Deltasone) and methylprednisolone (Medrol). An injectable steroid is triamcinolone (Aristocort).

OTHER THERAPIES ON THE HORIZON

Researchers are currently developing a new approach to allergies, using medication that is currently used for asthma patients. This is the administration of a humanized monoclonal anti-IgE antibody omalizumab (Xolair). This product seems to give patients with allergic rhinitis relief. However, it is very expensive at this time and is indicated only for severe asthma. Side effects include injection-site reaction, viral infections, upper-respiratory infections, sinusitis, headaches, and sore throat. Although rare, anaphylaxis can occur.

Treating Your Allergies for the Long Term: Immunization Therapy

All of the medications listed earlier are meant to control allergy symptoms. Allergy desensitization (immunotherapy) via allergy shot administration is a safe and highly effective way to relieve and/or eliminate allergic symptoms. In fact, allergen immunotherapy is the only form of therapy that will actually alter your body's immune response to allergens. In addition, it has been shown that this therapy may prevent the onset of asthma and even the onset of new allergies. Immunotherapy has also been shown to reduce medication usage and increase pulmonary function in asthmatics.

After careful allergy testing, an allergist can provide a formulation for your specific needs. A serum is created using purified extracts of the allergen and is administered as shots in the allergist's office. The shots are given weekly for approximately the first 6 months. The dose is increased each week until the final maintenance dose is reached, which can be significantly more concentrated than the initial dose. Once the maintenance dose is reached, the allergy shots can begin to be given less frequently. Monthly shots are continued for a period of 3 to 5 years. This time line for the shots is just an approximation and depends on the allergist's philosophy and the degree of severity of the allergy.

Although it is rare, an allergic reaction to the shots can occur at any time. This is why it is mandatory not only that the shots are administered in an allergist's office but that the patient remains in the office for 20 minutes after the injection.

Allergen immunotherapy should be considered for patients who continue to have moderate to severe symptoms despite therapy, who require systemic corticosteroids, who have an inadequate response to the recommended doses of nasal corticosteroids, or who have co-existing conditions such as sinusitis, asthma, or both.

SUBLINGUAL THERAPY

Allergen immunotherapy can also be administered by placing drops of the extract sublingually (under your tongue). Although mild oral and sublingual itching occurs, there have been no reports of systemic reactions to this therapy. The rarity of systemic reactions suggests that this therapy is safer than traditional allergy shots. However, the efficacy of sublingual therapy is apparently less than that of subcutaneous immunotherapy.

Sublingual immunotherapy is available only in certain centers in the United States because there is no commercial production available at this time.

Food Allergies

Another category of allergies is allergic reactions to specific foods. Allergies to food can cause skin reactions like hives and eczema. As well, the food allergens can cause swollen lips and upper- and lower-respiratory symptoms like allergic rhinitis and asthma.

Food allergies are more common in people who have other allergies. Food allergies have been witnessed since the beginning of time and can be fatal. At present, the only treatment for food allergies is complete avoidance.

Food allergies are often misunderstood and confused with other food-related sensitivities, including the following. Adverse reactions to foods and additives are non–life-threatening reactions to foods ingested. For example, some people have a strong reaction to monosodium glutamate (MSG), a chemically produced flavor enhancer often found in Chinese restaurant food (otherwise known as Kwok syndrome). After eating these foods, some people develop headaches, aching muscles in the face and head, or a tingly sensation. This is a reaction, but not an allergic phenomenon.

Food allergy or hypersensitivity to a food refers to a true allergic reaction involving the immune system. An example is hives caused by eating shrimp. Most often the substance causing the allergic reaction is a protein.

Food anaphylaxis is a true allergy involving IgE and can be fatal. The symptoms caused by the release of histamine and other inflammatory mediators include hives, throat swelling, a drop in blood pressure, wheezing, and abdominal cramping. Tree nuts, peanuts, and shellfish are the most common agents leading to anaphylaxis, but you can also develop a food allergy to any food group, including fruits, vegetables, dairy, and grains. There is a similar reaction without IgE involvement called anaphylactoid, meaning that it resembles anaphylaxis but without the IgE involvement. The most common agent that produces this type of reaction is the strawberry.

Metabolic food reactions/food intolerance occurs if you are unable to properly digest certain foods. Milk and milk products are common foods that cause this type of reaction, defined as lactose intolerance. This reaction is not an immune-mediated reaction. These people develop stomach cramps and diarrhea because they lack an enzyme known as lactase, which digests lactose sugar in milk. This is not an allergy.

Food poisoning is a reaction to a bacteria or a parasite, or possibly a reaction to a chemical in a food. This usually causes nausea and/or vomiting, diarrhea, and can cause fever. Food poisoning usually resolves itself within 24 hours.

A chemical reaction can be caused by an ingredient in a food. For example, many people are adversely affected by caffeine. They notice that when they eat chocolate or coffee they can become hyper and suffer from insomnia. The reaction to sugar is more controversial: It has been shown to affect some children by increasing their hyperactivity and/or anxiety. There has been a direct correlation to sugar and adrenaline in some of these people, but the reason is not clear. This response is not linked to an allergic reaction.

Allergic reaction to medication is a true allergic reaction, classified with food allergies because the medicine is ingested. Many people are allergic to medications as common as aspirin and some types of penicillin. It is important to keep careful records of medications that have caused true allergic reactions, including hives, throat swelling or closure, and wheezing. It is often difficult to discern a true medicine allergy from an adverse reaction.

CAID AND FOOD IRRITANTS

While true food allergies can be severe enough to cause anaphylaxis, many foods irritate the sinus system enough to cause discomfort. For example, milk products are known to increase mucus production and change its consistency, thereby exacerbating sinusitis. Alcohol consumption can make some people's sinus conditions flare: Their nasal and sinus membranes swell and polyp formation can occur. This swelling causes significant obstruction, mucus stagnation, and infection.

Allergies and Gastroesophageal Reflux Disease (GERD)

Perennial and seasonal allergies can affect not only your sinuses but your digestive system as well. The symptoms of GERD are not truly allergic but they can be related to a direct result of the allergic response. We know that allergies can cause gastroesophageal irritation stemming from the allergies themselves, which can cause GERD. We also know that allergy causes flare-ups of sinus problems, and that sinus problems cause a flare-up of GERD. People have demonstrated this connection, even though the exact scientific analysis has not been documented.

It is also interesting to note that the body is thought to be instinctively turned off to certain foods that may cause adverse digestive symptoms. Think for a moment about what foods you never eat and what foods you eat daily. The foods you avoid may in fact cause either an allergic response, GERD, or laryngopharyngeal reflux disease (LPRD). However, you may not realize that you are eating these foods if they appear as an ingredient in a processed, packaged, or prepared food, or a food that may be cooked at a friend's house or restaurant.

It is important to keep a food diary of foods that you think you either have an allergic reaction to or cause GERD, so that you can definitively determine your problem. Sharing this information with your allergist is an important step toward better health.

Chemical Sensitivities and Airborne Irritants

Airborne irritants are found in pollution. Although it has been known for some time, the latest research shows the dramatic effects pollution can have on the body. For example, car exhaust and irritants in the air can cause people who suffer from allergies to have similar reactions when exposed, even though they are not actually allergic to these pollutants. There is evidence that pollutants and irritants may play a role by increasing nasal responsiveness to environmental allergens. Furthermore, it has been shown that exposure to high levels of pollution may lead to asthma.

Are Allergies on the Rise?

Between 40 and 45 million Americans—about 15–20 percent of the population—have some type of allergy, most of which surface during infancy or childhood. The allergic march is a progression of symptoms that most often occurs in children. The first part of the march is atopic dermatitis, or scaly, itchy skin. About 75 percent of children who have atopic dermatitis go on to develop allergic rhinitis or hay fever, and about 50 percent of children with hay fever go on to develop asthma.

Food allergies also are increasing in children. Statistics show that food allergies affect 3.5–4 percent of the U.S. population. In the 1980s, it was estimated at about 0.5 percent. The prevalence of peanut allergies in the United States has about doubled since the mid-1990s. There are many theories regarding this increase in the incidence of both environmental and food allergies. Certainly public awareness and improved technology have led to an increase in accurate diagnosis of allergies. But then there are environmental reasons as well. Some feel that modern life is too "clean." They hypothesize that as babies are exposed to less dirt, disease, bacteria, and viruses their immune systems aren't activated correctly. In effect, without something real to fight, their immune system goes crazy, attacking things that aren't really dangerous, things like dust, peanuts, wheat, and even itself—which can lead to autoimmune diseases such as type 1 diabetes. This theory is called the hygiene hypothesis.

One study in Germany right after the reunification found that children in the former East Germany had fewer allergies than those in the former West Germany. Children in East Germany went into day-care centers at very young ages, where they proceeded to give each other lots of colds. It was theorized that having the diseases protected them against allergies, because their immune systems had something real to fight.

Some physicians believe that there may be some concrete steps parents can take to prevent the development of allergies in children. Although more research is required, it appears that these steps may help decrease the severity and/or likelihood that your child will develop allergies:

1. **Breast-feed for at least the first 4–6 months** of a child's life to help prevent allergies.
2. **Don't smoke.** There's universal agreement and numerous studies that being exposed to secondhand smoke increases asthma rates.
3. **Don't be afraid to expose your children to other children.** The constant runny nose and colds of the day-care center or school are actually a good substitute for the colds passed between the larger numbers of children that most families used to have. Researchers now say that exposure to the common illnesses of childhood helps fine-tune a child's immune system. Without such exposure, it sometimes strikes out at the wrong things, causing allergies and autoimmune disorders.
4. **Don't have peanuts or products containing peanuts in the house until your child is at least 1.** Children can be sensitized to peanuts simply by having someone else in the house eat them. A British study found that families with peanuts in the house have a higher rate of peanut allergy compared with households

with no peanut exposure. However, the question about whether pregnant women should avoid peanuts is not answered. Some researchers believe that prenatal exposure can trigger sensitivity; others believe that it can protect the child.

5. **If you're going to have dogs and cats, get them before you have children.** Research has shown that when there is a dog or a cat in the house when a baby arrives, the child gains some protection against later developing animal allergies. This appears to work with dogs slightly more than cats. Getting a pet even a few months later doesn't seem to have the same effect.

CHAPTER 6

MANAGING ASTHMA

Asthma is one of the most serious, if not life-threatening, symptoms of chronic airway-digestive inflammatory disease (CAID). There are millions of people who are affected by asthma, ranging from the very young to the very old, crossing ethnic barriers and socioeconomic groups. In the United States, asthma is the number one killer of children.

The symptoms of asthma directly affect our ability to breathe, which we often take for granted. If you have ever experienced an asthma attack or have witnessed a child or a friend suffering from asthma, then you know full well how scary it can be.

An asthma attack can be caused by something as benign as cold air or exertion. Allergies and drugs (such as aspirin or nonsteroidal anti-inflammatory drugs like Advil or Motrin) have been linked to asthma, as has stress. For people with asthma, the main goal of therapy is the prevention of chronic asthma symptoms so they can maintain a good quality of life without disruption—in school or work—and without frequent emergency room visits or hospitalizations.

Asthma is defined as a reversible constriction of the airways. In most instances, this causes wheezing. However, you can have asthma without wheezing, and there are other disorders that cause wheezing unrelated to asthma.

Understanding the Respiratory System

Asthma affects the functioning of the lungs and the entire respiratory system. As discussed in Chapter 1, the nose is the portal to our body's airway, allowing us to breathe clean, filtered, and humidified air. Once air is processed by the sinuses, it moves toward the lungs through the trachea (Diagram 13, page 32). The trachea divides into two branches, or bronchi, each feeding into one of the lungs. Within each lung, the bronchi further divide into thousands of smaller branches, forming the bronchial tree. Each branch is surrounded by rings of muscles that constrict and relax in response to various stimuli as we breathe, allowing air to flow freely.

The air we inhale then travels to the tips of the bronchial tree and eventually reaches the alveolus, where the exchange of oxygen and carbon dioxide takes place among the network of blood vessels that surround it. The bronchi and alveoli are lined with their own mucous membranes, which perform the same filtering and humidifying functions as the ones in our nose and mouth.

What Happens During an Asthma Attack?

During an asthma attack, the muscles surrounding the bronchi tighten, significantly reducing the size of the bronchi (Diagram 18). This is referred to as acute (sudden) airway obstruction. Meanwhile, the mucous membrane that lines the bronchi and alveoli begins to swell and produce more mucus, further obstructing the bronchi. This inflammation can occur as a response to various stimuli; changes in the structure and function of this lining dramatically affect the severity of an asthma attack. When the airways become severely narrowed and obstructed, there is very limited air flow. The efforts for inhaling must increase to get the proper amount of air into the lung.

Due to the difficulty in moving the air in and out of the lungs, all the muscles connected to the respiratory system are involuntarily called

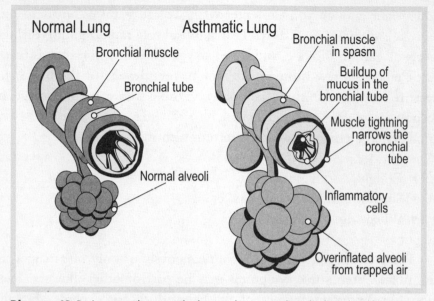

Diagram 18 During an asthma attack, the muscles surrounding the bronchi tighten, significantly reducing the size of the bronchi.

into action. It is common to see someone during an acute attack using "abdominal breathing," in which abdominal muscles are used to suck in more air. The ribs and the abdominal muscles will become concave, and the neck muscles will rise and fall with each breath. During milder attacks, these signs may be more subtle, yet the sufferer is still literally fighting to take a breath.

The mucus clogging the bronchial tubes becomes thickened and infected, causing chronic cough and shortness of breath. The lungs will automatically begin to wheeze. The wheezing is the high-pitched sound of the air pushing through the bronchi as it tries to get to the lungs. In rare instances, asthma symptoms can also include chest pain, hyperventilation, and spitting blood.

An acute attack is literally exhausting, and the sufferer will quickly become tired and reduce his or her rate of respiration. If you are experiencing a severe asthma attack, you can feel as if you were suffocating. In fact, that is what is happening. When the breathing passageways clamp down tight enough you can enter what we call status asthmaticus; and there is essentially no airflow. This can lead to a rapid buildup of high levels of carbon dioxide, and lower oxygen levels in the bloodstream. All it takes is a few moments of low oxygen levels for the brain and heart to stop functioning, causing irreversible stroke, brain damage, or coma.

There is a classic triad of symptoms seen with asthma:

- Cough
- Shortness of breath
- Wheezing

These symptoms may occur simultaneously or only one may occur at a time. Often, these symptoms may be part of other illnesses. Even more confusing, an absence of wheezing does not exclude an acute asthma attack. When the airways become severely narrowed and obstructed, the air flow is so limited that wheezing does not occur. On the other hand, wheezing can be seen with other disorders. This can happen if there is a foreign body aspirated into the lung or with the presence of mucus in the airway by the vocal cords or in the nose. It is, therefore, very important for you to relay your symptoms to your doctor so that he or she can make an accurate diagnosis.

CAID and Asthma

Many of the same triggers for CAID can also prompt an asthma attack. Sinus disease is now recognized as a leading factor in respiratory illnesses and is known to actually worsen asthma. The sinuses are the filters that clean the air we breathe: It, therefore, makes sense that breathing dirty air will irritate the lungs. Postnasal drip alone is a common cause of asthmatic flare-up leading to wheezing. Asthma also tends to occur with people who can't breathe through their nose because of constant blockage. For example, people with nasal polyps often suffer from asthma. But in the worst-case scenario, these people suffer from nasal polyps, asthma, and allergy to aspirin or nonsteroidal anti-inflammatory drugs such as Motrin. This disease process with the triad of symptoms is called Samter's triad, or triad asthma.

An asthma attack can also be triggered by many of the same irritants that affect CAID sufferers. Smoke, pollution, allergens (environmental as well as food), chemicals, and particular scents are all culprits, as well as infections caused by viruses, fungi or bacteria.

Gastroesophageal reflux disease/laryngopharyngeal reflux disease (GERD/LPRD) is also connected to asthma. Acid reflux from the stomach can enter the lungs when the muscle that normally closes the passage between the esophagus and the stomach is relaxed. When a person lies down, the acid can pass through this juncture and into the esophagus and into the windpipe (trachea). In the windpipe, irritation by the reflux causes the contraction of the bronchial muscles, which begins the asthma attack.

Your allergies can trigger your asthma as a symptom, just the same way as they make your eyes water or nose run. However, asthma symptoms are far more dangerous than your typical runny nose. I have seen mild to no allergies in people with severe asthma and I have seen severe allergies with minimal or no asthma in others.

Jay is a 25-year-old patient of mine who tested negative to allergies, yet he suffers from chronic sinus infections and asthma. Working together, Jay and I were able to determine that his CAID was causing his asthma to flare. When his sinuses flare his asthma flares; and as this happens, his GERD starts acting up. As the postnasal drip worsens, he starts wheezing, belching, and coughing. The good news is that when you treat your CAID symptoms regularly, you will find that you can also keep your asthma and GERD under control. Once I started Jay on the right regimen of holistic and prescriptive treatments, he was feeling better and breathing much easier.

Defining Asthma Symptoms and Conditions

Based on the intensity of the symptoms, asthma is classified as one of the following:

- **Mild intermittent asthma.** People with this condition experience symptoms less than twice a week, with no more than two nocturnal awakenings per month, meaning that they are awakened from sleep because of difficulty breathing. Typically, those in this category develop symptoms when being exposed to a triggering factor such as allergens or pollutants. Others develop their symptoms when they have been exposed to an upper-respiratory infection or during strenuous physical exercise, more commonly called exercise-induced asthma.

- **Mild persistent asthma.** People with this condition experience symptoms more than twice a week with more than two nighttime awakenings per month.

- **Moderate persistent asthma.** This description is given to people who have daily symptoms, with exacerbations that affect the quality of life at least once a week, meaning that not only do they need to take their medication daily, they are also debilitated by the disease. If not treated properly, this group is at high risk to suffer long-term, irreversible damage to the lungs.

- **Acute exacerbations of acute asthma.** Acute asthma refers to the actual sudden attack. During an acute attack, patients will feel the following symptoms: the inability to lie down owing severe shortness of breath, the use of multiple groups of muscles to ease breathing, cold sweats, and anxiety. During an acute attack, it is common to see a period of mild improvement followed by rapid deterioration. If you or someone you know is experiencing these symptoms, go immediately to the nearest emergency room to seek treatment. Because of the major risks of complications, it is common to remain in the hospital for observation and treatment until steady improvement is noted.

WHEN IT'S NOT ASTHMA

Wheezing and shortness of breath can occur even if you do not have asthma. For example, a bronchial infection, known as bronchitis, might make you feel as if you were suffering from asthma. During bronchitis, the bronchial tubes are chronically constricted and partially or totally blocked by the large amount of mucus produced by the inflamed lining. These features often are mistaken as asthma, and the treatment you would receive is almost exactly the same as what would be prescribed for an asthma attack. The exception is that for bacterial bronchitis, you would also be treated with antibiotics. However, with proper medication, and reversal of the triggering factors, asthma should be completely reversible: Your breathing will immediately return to normal. With a bronchial infection, especially if it becomes chronic, the condition can be controlled but is not reversible. For an acute bronchitis, treatment will resolve the problem but it will not occur immediately. Therefore, if you find that you are wheezing without the presence of other asthma symptoms including shortness of breath, you should discuss this symptom with your doctor.

Chronic bronchitis, which is a subset of chronic obstructive pulmonary disease (COPD), is also often confused with asthma. This disease is directly linked to cigarette smoking and pollution. A chronic smoker or someone exposed to significant air pollution can develop major permanent destruction of the air passages in the lungs. For these patients, the major bronchial tubes are so damaged by the chronic bronchitis process that they do constrict and can fill with excessive mucus. Asthma medications will have limited, if any effect for improving the shortness of breath caused by this disease.

Unfortunately, it is not uncommon for someone to be told by one doctor that he or she has asthma, only to be told a month later by another doctor that it's emphysema. The two can look the same, although emphysema is not reversible, whereas asthma is.

Decoding My Problem

Asthma symptoms should not be taken lightly. Review your results from the asthma portion of the CAID Quiz (p. 72). Locate your score so that you can define your next course of action. Follow the guidelines as listed here:

- Any asthma score greater than 5 should be treated by a physician.
- If you also suffer from other CAID symptoms, you need to see an ear, nose, and throat (ENT) doctor who specializes in treating CAID, or at least has an understanding of the relationship between sinus disease and asthma.

Because of the connection between the nose and the lungs, people with asthma are often directed to be treated by a team of physicians, including an otolaryngologist (ENT), allergist, and/or a pulmonologist. Very often it is the ENT who leads the team of specialists.

A Visit with a Physician

A careful history, a comprehensive physical examination, and pulmonary function tests, should help a physician narrow down your complaints. Make sure to relay all prior episodes of asthma or lung problems, allergies, family history of asthma or allergies, and triggering factors that you have decoded.

The pulmonary function tests are designed to diagnose various lung diseases. The simplest test involves breathing through a tube into a computerized system. This test, called spirometry, measures the forcefulness of your inhalations and exhalations (Diagram 19). Spirometry is easy to perform, and most doctors who treat asthma have the instrument available in the office. This test generates some numeric values to rate your forcefulness. It also creates a graph, called a flow-volume loop, which is recorded by the computer. The loop above the vertical axis

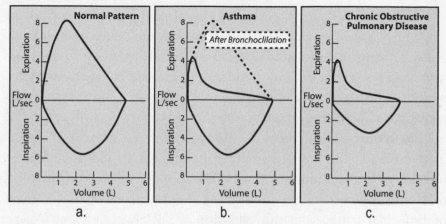

Diagram 19 These spirometric graphs show various stages of asthma and pulmonary disease.

represents the exhalation and the loop below represents inhalation. The shape of the loop is specific for various lung diseases. For example, the first loop in 19 shows normal breathing. This shape is also shown for people with asthma when they are not flaring, because their lungs will typically look normal when they are not experiencing an attack.

Spirometry can be performed in two stages: the first stage to diagnose and the second to assess any therapeutic effect of the medications. The second stage is done after medication has been given to dilate the bronchial tubes. If asthma is present, then the loop should return to normal after the treatment. This is shown in the second part of the diagram: The asthmatic loop is superimposed on the normal loop, which shows the response to treatment. If there is a fixed disease like emphysema, there will be no improvement. Remember that you can have a mixed pattern, which makes testing more complicated. The third loop shows changes on the top and bottom of the loop, consistent with COPD, bronchitis, and emphysema.

Pulmonary function tests help diagnose more subtle forms of asthma that occur during exertion only, or as a result of various stimulants. In a subset of bronchial asthma called exercise-induced asthma, spirometry is done after a provocation test either by exercise in a controlled environment or by inhalation of chemical substances known to induce symptoms.

Pulse oximetry can be performed by placing a device on your finger, which is used to measure the arterial oxygen concentration in the blood. During an acute asthmatic attack, as less air flows into the lungs, less oxygen is extracted and circulates within the bloodstream. A low oxygen concentration is very dangerous as it may cause heart attacks, strokes, or respiratory collapse.

Blood tests can also be performed to check the amount of oxygen in your blood. This is called an arterial blood gas. In addition, there are blood tests to determine the level of eosinophils or other white blood cells in your blood. A high count of eosinophils is one of the hallmarks of bronchial asthma, but this elevation is not always present. Allergy testing may also be performed to see if there is an allergic component to the attacks.

Chest X-rays are usually normal between attacks. During an acute attack of asthma, due to excessive trapping of air in the lungs, the appearance is hyperinflated. Chest X-rays can also help exclude pneumonia, which could be the triggering factor of an acute asthma attack.

Medical Treatment Options

Asthma can be completely controlled through the proper and consistent use of medication. The type of proper medical treatment depends on what kind of asthma you have, and the severity of your symptoms. Treatment is divided into two protocols: long-term control or maintenance for each of the various types of asthma and quick relief during acute exacerbations.

LONG-TERM AND MAINTENANCE TREATMENT PROTOCOLS

Treatment of mild, intermittent asthma may involve intermittent use of inhaled beta-antagonist agents. If you have exercise-induced asthma, your treatment should be administered 10–20 minutes before beginning physical activity. In addition, inhaled chromones can be used before exposure. This will act as a preventive treatment: they are not useful once the symptoms develop.

Treatment of mild, persistent asthma begins by adding an anti-inflammatory agent, such as inhaled corticosteroids (ICSs), to your medications. Long-acting inhaled beta-antagonists can be used in this stage as a component of the treatment protocol but should not be used alone. A leukotriene modifying agent, such as Zyflo, should be considered if your asthma symptoms are not well controlled with the inhaled corticosteroids alone. If you have been diagnosed with mild, persistent asthma, you might be a good candidate for allergy testing. If your testing is positive, then you should be treated for your allergies.

The treatment for moderate persistent asthma includes inhaled corticosteroids, prescribed at a higher dosage, along with short acting beta-antagonists. The ICS dose should be reduced if the symptoms are well controlled. But if the symptoms persist after a few weeks of intense ICS therapy, a second agent, such as theophylline or leukotriene should be added.

When you suffer from an acute severe asthma attack, rapid reversal of asthma symptoms is accomplished with multiple doses of inhaled, short-acting beta-antagonists, including Albuterol. At times, it is necessary to administer continuous nebulization with a compressor to obtain relief. To combat bronchial inflammation, intravenous or oral corticosteroids are often used, although they can take up to 6 hours to begin working. Antibiotics are used if an infection is suspected or proven to be a triggering factor of the asthma. Lastly, oxygen is given to correct the low oxygen levels. Magnesium sulfate can also be given intravenously as it has a bronchodilator effect.

Delivering Asthma Medications

Because asthma attacks can occur with a quick onset, the best way to deliver medication is often by inhaling it. Inhaled medications relax the muscles around the bronchial tubes so that air can flow freely. Inhaled medications can be delivered in three distinct ways. The first is via a small compressor called a nebulizer. Liquid medication is poured into a chamber that is connected with tubing to both the nebulizer and a face mask or sucking tube. A tube or mask is placed in front of the face, and the nebulizer forces the liquid medication into a constant gaseous stream so that it can be inhaled. The nebulizer is the best way to deliver this type of medication. Unlike the older models, the newer models are light, quiet, and portable. You can even use it in a car by plugging it into the cigarette lighter.

The second method for inhaling medications is through the use of a metered dose inhaler (MDI) (Diagram 20). An MDI can fit easily into a pocket, so that you can take your medication wherever you go. The efficiency of the treatment is enhanced by the use of a spacer (Diagram 21). This is a tube with a mouth mask on one side and a connective port for an MDI on the other. The MDI releases a spray of medication into the spacer, which traps the medication from the MDI until the user draws it into his or her lungs by inhaling. The spacer also ensures that all of the medication is delivered without any loss in open space. It also reduces the side effects of some medications by limiting the amount of the medication that is deposited in the mouth and in the back of the throat. An MDI is smaller than a nebulizer and does not require a power source.

How to Use an MDI

Here's the most effective way to use an MDI:

1. Shake the canister before each treatment.
2. Slowly breathe out all the air in your lungs.
3. Remove the cap and place the inhaler in your mouth with your lips around the mouth piece.
4. Press the activator once.
5. Take one slow, deep breath until you fully inflate your lungs.
6. Hold your breath for 5–10 seconds.
7. Breathe out.
8. Repeat the entire process in 3–5 minutes.

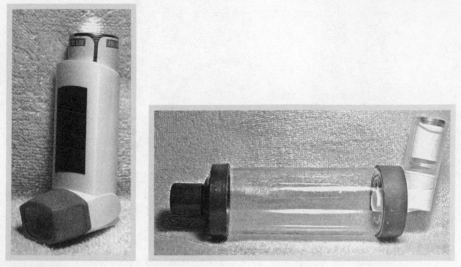

Diagram 20   **Diagram 21**

A metered dose inhaler (Diagram 20) is especially effective when used in conjunction with a spacer (Diagram 21).

Dry Powder Inhalers

Inhaled medication can also be dispensed in a dry powder form. For some, the inhalation technique is easier than the MDI: You do not have to synchronize your breathing with the pressure of the inhaler. For powders, the medication is released by your inhalation effort, known as breath activated. A commonly used dry powder inhaler is Advair. This combines two medications: a long-acting beta-agonist and a corticosteroid powder. This combination should not be used as a rescue medication during an acute attack, as it has a long onset of action (Diagram 22).

LONG-TERM MEDICATIONS

Inhaled Corticosteroids

ICSs play an important role in the management of chronic asthma. Studies have shown that if used regularly, the ICSs reduce the frequency of the symptoms, reduce the need for rescue inhalers, reduce the risk

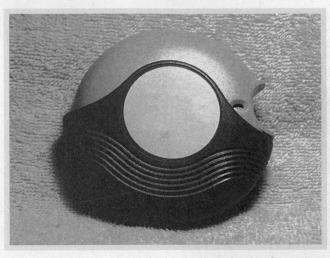

Diagram 22 A dry powder inhaler can also be used and is often easier to operate. With this device you do not have to synchronize your breathing with the pressure of the inhaler.

of serious complications, lower the rate of hospital admissions, and improve the quality of life overall.

A common side effect is the development of an oral fungal infection called thrush. The risk of this can be reduced by using a spacer with an MDI, and rinsing your mouth immediately after the medication has been administered. ICSs have less systemic side effects compared with the oral steroids due to the fact that the medication is delivered to the lungs with only minimal absorption into the bloodstream. However, some studies have shown significant bone loss in patients using high doses of ICS.

Commonly prescribed ICSs
Fluticasone (Flovent)
Budesonide (Pulmicort)
Beclomethasone (Beclovent, Vanceril, Becloforte, Qvar)
Triamcinolone (Azmacort)

Leukotriene Receptor Antagonists

A new class of medication used in the treatment of bronchial asthma is leukotriene receptor antagonists. This medication blocks the release of the chemical compounds that are normally released by the inflammatory mucous membranes in the lung during the acute phases of asthma. Those chemical compounds, if not blocked, have a powerful constricting effect on the bronchial tubes. Sole therapy with this medication is reserved primarily for treatment of mild persistent asthma. It may also be added on to other therapies, such as inhaled corticosteroids, in more severe asthma. It has no beneficial effects in the treatment of acute, severe asthma attacks. The first generation in this class includes montelukast (Singulair) and zafirlukast (Accolate).

The latest agent in this class, Zyflo, has been shown to have an effect on a higher level of the inflammatory cascade. Studies have shown that when used regularly, it reduces the need for rescue inhalers, reduces the frequency of nighttime symptoms, and can improve the overall quality of life.

Inhaled Cromones (Mast Cell Stabilizers)

Mast cell stabilizers act by reducing the inflammation of the bronchial tubes and seem to be effective in mild asthma. They are also found to be more effective in children than in adults. These medicines include Cromolyn and Nedocromil. To gain the most benefit, do not miss doses. Side effects are minimal, but include the following:

- **Oral inhalation.** Sore throat and dry mouth, which may be managed by frequent mouth care, sucking harder on the MDI, sucking sugar-free candy, or chewing sugar-free gum.
- **Nasal.** Nasal irritation.

Anticholinergics

Anticholinergics block the chemical that causes the contractions of bronchial tubes as well as excessive mucus production. Ipatropium bromide is a commonly used anticholinergic. It may be used alone or in combination with a fast-acting, emergency medication like albuterol. Some studies have shown that the combination of the two drugs (available in one MDI) increases bronchial dilation better than if either is used alone. This treatment should be used for long-term maintenance of asthma.

QUICK-RELIEF, OR EMERGENCY MEDICATIONS

Quick-relief medications relax the muscles around the bronchial tubes so that air can flow freely through them. As noted earlier, these medications are called bronchodilators or beta-agonists because they connect rapidly to beta-receptors, causing them to work. These agents work well but act only for a short period of time. The most common agent in this category is albuterol (Proventil, Volmax); other common prescriptions are levalbuterol (Xopenex) and pirbuterol (Maxair). The advantage of the latter agent is that it is more selective and causes fewer side effects, such as palpitations and rapid heart beat. Its effects last for 6–8 hours, whereas albuterol lasts for 4–6 hours. During severe acute attacks, it is often necessary to give these medications via continuous nebulization over a long period of time.

Salmeterol (Serevent) is a longer-acting inhaled beta-agonist, but it is still not a preventative medication. It can last up to 12 hours, so it is primarily used to control symptoms during the night. It should not be used during an acute attack. This product is no longer available alone, but is available as a combination medicine.

ORAL CORTICOSTEROIDS

Steroids in an oral or intravenous form are used to treat a range of asthma attacks. Their role is to reduce the inflammation of the bronchial tube's lining, thus reducing the accumulation of mucus and clogging of the airways. The side effects of oral steroids are serious, as discussed in earlier chapters. However, a single treatment regimen of steroids is relatively safe. An intravenous dose of steroids should be administered for the quick relief treatment of an acute asthma attack.

Theophylline

Theophylline was considered the work horse of asthma therapy until a few years ago. Its benefits have been overshadowed by its significant side effects (racing heartbeat and palpitations) and its interaction with other medications. These side effects are worsened by caffeine (tea, coffee, cola, and chocolate) intake. Use is also cautioned if you have peptic ulcer disease, hyperthyroidism, seizure disorders, high blood pressure, or cardiac arrhythmias. Your blood levels should be regularly monitored if you are taking this medication.

OXYGEN

During an acute attack, it is necessary to administer oxygen continuously until the flare-up is completely over. As described earlier, during an asthma flare-up, your oxygen levels can drop considerably. Oxygen should be administered only under a doctor's direct supervision.

ASTHMA MEDICATIONS DURING PREGNANCY

Women with asthma used to be discouraged from becoming pregnant, but advances in medication have made pregnancy extremely possible. Yet like all other aspects of pregnancy, it can change the natural course of asthma. Asthma symptoms can worsen, improve, or remain unchanged. The general principles of asthma therapy can be followed during pregnancy, with these guidelines:

- Inhaled selective beta-adrenergic drugs—generally safe during pregnancy
- Theophylline—safe during pregnancy but requires close monitoring
- ICS—considered safe during pregnancy
- Ipratropium—considered safe during pregnancy
- Corticosteroids—given orally or intravenously, low risk of complications; given only when clinically necessary (Possible fetal complications: congenital malformations, low birth weight, and

adrenal gland malfunction; maternal risks: diabetes or hypertension)

- Leukotriene modifiers—have not been tested on humans and generally discouraged
- Antihistamines for asthma that is allergy induced or decongestants used for corresponding congestion—can be used but only when absolutely necessary and under a doctor's care

Children and Asthma

Children usually experience complete remission from asthma more frequently than adults do. Between 30 and 70 percent of children who develop asthma either improve or are totally asymptomatic after the onset of puberty. Asthma appears to be more severe in girls than in boys. Furthermore, a small subgroup of children with asthma is linked to maternal smoking. It is interesting that recent studies have shown that those children who have asthma may be at a decreased risk of developing brain cancer later in life.

Asthma medications can be prescribed to children at a very young age. Children suffering from asthma may be nebulized with albuterol, even as infants. If your child exhibits any asthma symptoms, see a doctor immediately, and have your child tested for allergies as well as asthma. The earlier children are treated, the more likely it is that they will grow out of their symptoms.

Lifestyle Changes

Asthma related to allergies and CAID can be controlled, and often prevented, through avoidance and education. If you can recognize your triggers, as well as your trigger symptoms, you will be able to control your asthma through early use of your medication.

The first step is to create an asthma action plan with your doctor. This includes knowing when to take your medication and when to avoid your triggers, especially if they are allergens or irritants.

One invaluable tool for people with asthma is the peak flow meter, a handy, noninvasive way to assess the otherwise subjective signs such as cough, wheezing, shortness of breath. Peak flow meters can be purchased at any pharmacy and come with easy to understand instructions and a diary to record daily values. Some of them are small enough to be carried in a pocket or purse. Digital peak flow meters are also available. One such product, the PIKo is able to store all of the measurements inside a computer chip. A physician is able to download these to a computer and analyze your asthma trends. This can help guide therapeutic decisions by your physician.

To use a peak flow meter (Diagram 23), you need to take a deep breath and blow into it. This records your average level of forcefulness, called your "personal best score." You can compare this score to how you feel right after taking your daily medications and whenever you feel the onset of an attack. Each peak flow meter has three value zones:

Green (okay) zone   80–100 % of personal best
Yellow (caution) zone   50–80% of personal best
Red (danger) zone   <50% of personal best

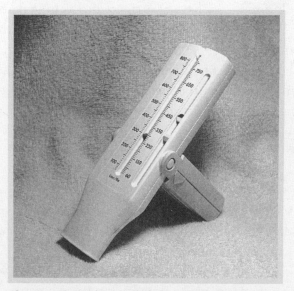

Diagram 23 The data gained from a peak flow meter can be used by your physician to help guide therapeutic decisions.

Your personal best value is as individual as you are. It depends on your age, height, and gender. However, your personal best score should fall within the green zone.

Surgical Treatments

There are no surgical treatments that can control asthma symptoms, but for patients who suffer from both sinus disease that requires surgery and asthma, I have found that these patients report that their asthma flares less often after they have had sinus surgery. In the past, sinus surgery was not recommended for those with asthma for fear that these patients would stop breathing during surgery. This limitation was thought to be caused by the large amount of bleeding encountered during traditional techniques of sinus surgery: Blood could be aspirated into the lungs, and the subsequent nasal packing could potentially cause an asthma flare-up.

The latest endoscopic techniques have limited the amount of bleeding during surgery. Packing is not needed in almost all cases, and aspiration does not occur or is insignificant. In addition, older general anesthetic techniques may have contributed to asthma flare-ups after sinus surgery. Today, surgery is performed under local anesthesia with sedation and there is no general anesthesia required in most instances. However, when general anesthesia is needed, the techniques and agents used today are better than they were in the past. Most asthma patients who had sinus surgery, report that their asthma improved after surgery.

CHAPTER 7

TREATING GERD AND LPRD ONCE AND FOR ALL

Gastroesophageal reflux disease (GERD) and laryngopharyngeal reflux disease (LPRD) make up the last branch of chronic airway-digestive inflammatory disease (CAID). When we swallow, food and liquids travel through the esophagus and land in the stomach, where stomach acids help the digestive process. Within the esophagus are two constricting muscles: the lower esophageal sphincter and the upper esophageal sphincter. During normal swallowing, these rings of muscle open and close at the precise moment that food passes through the esophagus. When the lower esophageal sphincter is not functioning properly, there is a backflow of stomach acid into the esophagus. This acid flow irritates the esophagus causing heartburn, a painful, burning sensation in the chest. If this happens, it can be a sign of GERD. Additionally, recent research reveals that the stomach enzyme pepsin causes damage to the airway-digestive membranes when it refluxes.

Those of us who experience GERD have a clear picture of how it feels. Typically, the profile of a GERD patient is someone who is sedentary; is slightly overweight; and has a history of burping, heartburn, and stomach pain, usually associated with meals. GERD sufferers often regurgitate their food, particularly at night, which can cause chronic coughing. This symptom is usually a clue that the GERD complications are reaching beyond the esophagus. When the upper esophageal sphincter doesn't function correctly, acid that has already flowed back into the esophagus enters the throat and voice box. When this happens, acidic material contacts the sensitive tissue at the back of the throat and even the back of the nasal airway—causing heartburn, sore throat, phlegm, postnasal drip, cough, choking, hoarseness, and/or CAID. This is known as LPRD. GERD and LPRD can occur separately or together.

Other symptoms of LPRD include a bitter taste in the back of the throat, which commonly occurs in the morning upon awakening, and the sensation of a lump or something stuck in the throat, which does not go away despite multiple swallowing attempts. Some adults may also experience a burning sensation in the throat. Others may find themselves with ear pain caused by inflammation of the throat; laryngitis caused by the inflammation of the voice box from the reflux; gingivitis, which is irritation and inflammation of the gums as a result of the acids burning the membranes around the teeth; nasal obstruction caused by the inflammation of the nasal membranes, resulting in nasal swelling; noisy breathing (stridor) caused by the inflammation and swelling around the airway; or bad breath (halitosis).

More than half of LPRD sufferers do not experience heartburn: The stomach acid does not stay in the esophagus long enough to irritate the esophagus and cause these symptoms. In LPRD, most of the damage to the esophagus and/or the throat caused by reflux that happens without you ever knowing it. The frequency and the contact time of the acid with mucous membranes in the pharynx is much greater than the contact with the esophagus. Compared to the esophagus, the mucous membranes in the voice box and the back of the throat are significantly more sensitive to the affects of stomach acids. Acid that passes quickly through the food pipe does not have a chance to irritate the area for too long. However, acid that pools in the throat and voice box will cause prolonged irritation, resulting in the symptoms of LPRD. For this reason, LPRD is often referred to as "silent GERD," and can be very difficult to diagnose.

Irritation in the voice box can lead to a laryngospasm, which means that the voice box contracts. This can be a very scary: It feels as if you were going to choke or suffocate. Some doctors believe that laryngospasm, GERD, and panic attacks are related. Worst of all, acids can enter the trachea and the lungs, where they can be even more damaging. These tissues will become irritated, leading to bronchitis and asthma. In patients who have bad asthma, this irritation can set off status asthmaticus, in which the lungs tighten up and you cannot get air. Status asthmaticus is rarely caused by reflux; but if it occurs, it can be life threatening.

Finally, 10–15 percent of patients who have chronic GERD can end up with histologic changes of the esophageal lining. This occurs in the lower esophagus. This disease is called Barrett's esophagus: In rare instances, the acids cause the normal lining of the esophagus to be replaced by the type of lining that is found in the stomach or intestine. When this membrane is continuously subjected to refluxing acid, esophageal cancer can develop. A gastroenterologist can make this diagnosis with an outpatient endoscopy and biopsy of the esophagus. For people found to have these changes, close monitoring of the esophagus is necessary. Furthermore, the refluxing acids can potentially cause ulcers in the esophagus. Although this is also rare, these ulcers can hemorrhage and perforate. For all of these reasons, it is very important to control severe reflux (Diagram 24).

GERD/LPRD and Sinus Disease

Recent scientific research indicates that acid reflux into the throat (pharynx) plays a role in the development of sinusitis in both children and adults. Although acid reflux usually does not reach all the way to the sinuses, it could induce inflammation of the sensitive nasal mucous membranes, thus blocking the sinuses. Patients with GERD or LPRD are also less likely to get relief from sinus surgery if their reflux is not addressed.

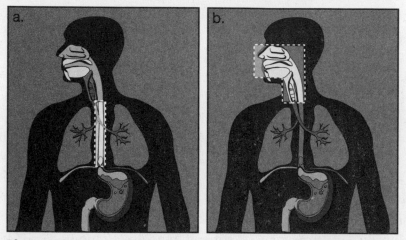

Diagram 24 a: In patients with GERD (left), the stomach contents back up (reflux) into the esophagus, causing heartburn or indigestion (esophagitis-inflammation of the esophagus). b: In patients with LPRD (right), the stomach acid does not stay in the esophagus long enough to cause heartburn, but instead travels to the larynx (voice box) and pharynx (throat) and nose and sinuses. Here the acids cause irritation and inflammation. The acids in the larynx can cause laryngospasm or can aspirate into the lungs. Some people suffer from both GERD and LPRD.

Unfortunately, the exact cause-and-effect mechanism of acid reflux and sinusitis has not yet been established. For example, postnasal drip can occur from inflammation of the nose by the stomach acids or it can be caused by chronic sinusitis. We also know that when postnasal drip lines the throat and the esophagus, it can cause reflux to worsen. I believe that this is secondary to the gag reflex but also that it may occur as a result of stimulation to the autonomic nervous system. Furthermore, older people often complain that when they eat, their nose runs. This is further evidence that there is a connection between the stomach and the nose. I believe that this is also via the autonomic nervous system. Last, when infection in the sinuses drips into the stomach, the infecting bacteria and fungus upset the normal balance of stomach organisms. The stomach reacts to this imbalance and this can potentially cause the reflux to act up.

Symptoms of LPRD, especially in children, can be difficult to diagnose. For sufferers with chronic sinusitis, the symptom of postnasal drip can make them feel the same way as those that suffer from LPRD. Or the symptoms can occur because of a combination of the two disease processes. For all of these reasons, I believe that GERD/LPRD is intimately related with sinus disease, and thus I include it within the definition of CAID.

As you start to understand each, you will also be able to decipher exactly what is acting up at all times and often can tell which came first. For example, when your sinuses are acting up, you can feel your nose get congested, and you begin to suffer from the usual sinus symptoms—postnasal drip, nasal discharge, cough, hoarseness, pressure, and headaches. When your GERD/LPRD is acting up by itself you can feel mild heartburn or begin to belch, expel gas, cough, or have a feeling of fullness in the throat. When they are both acting up, you can feel both sets of symptoms. Sometimes your sinuses can be the first to start, and you feel the postnasal drip and instinctively start swallowing and clearing your throat. Then you can find yourself belching, clearing your throat more, coughing, and your voice can become hoarse. When this occurs, you might want to jump out of your skin, especially when you are in public. It is impossible to attribute a cause for every symptom. In these cases, treatments should be focused toward both your sinuses and your stomach.

My patient Sandra ate a dinner of pasta with a glass or two of wine. About 20 minutes into the meal she began to feel congested. Her sinuses seemed to have acted up in response to both the carbohydrates and the alcohol. She began to feel postnasal drip in the back of her throat. When this happens, Sandra usually can't clear her throat, and she begins to cough. Her reflux also starts. Sandra notes that she will start belching and coughing and feel a slight heaviness in her chest. This description is consistent with someone experiencing full-blown GERD/LPRD caused by a sinus flare-up. Both the sinus flare-up and the GERD/LPRD appear to be related to carbohydrate and alcohol consumption. In other words, this becomes a vicious cycle, with the reflux causing more postnasal drip, creating more congestion and inflammation with more drip causing more reflux. However, once the sinus problem and the GERD/LPRD are treated, Sandra will return to normal.

It is interesting that another patient, Dane, a GERD sufferer, told me that he didn't realize his GERD was connected to sinus problems. He had been treated for years by various physicians and no one mentioned it. Dane told me that he went online and found a massive amount of literature on the connection between sinus disease and GERD. He was surprised that many people don't make a connection between these disorders. Unfortunately, the people who know best are the ones who suffer from these disease processes.

Silent GERD/LPRD

Sometimes you can experience a feeling in your throat with none of the usual symptoms of GERD—heartburn, indigestion, and reflux. For example, you may complain only of hoarseness. Others may complain of coughing fits or a feeling of fullness, making them want to clear their throat. Then there are the others that are experiencing bouts of laryngospasm. Still others may just suffer from occasional or chronic sore throat when their LPRD acts up. These are the more difficult cases to diagnose because their symptoms are not classic textbook. Often, these people jump from physician to physician without finding relief. Unless the physician and the patient are spending the time to analyze the problem, it will continue to be misdiagnosed. This is the reason why it is so important for you to speak your doctor's language.

Symptoms of LPRD
- Apnea—shortness of breath
- Aspiration pneumonia
- Asthma-like symptoms
- Bad/bitter taste in mouth (especially in morning)
- Bad breath (halitosis)

- Blockage of the breathing passage, laryngospasm
- Chronic cough
- Chronic nasal congestion
- Chronic throat irritation (sore throat)
- Chronic throat clearing, excessive mucus
- Constant sensation of a lump in the throat
- Cracking voice
- Dental caries
- Difficulty singing, especially with high notes
- Difficulty swallowing
- Ear pain
- Excessive phlegm in the throat
- Frequent laryngitis
- Gagging
- Gingivitis
- Heartburn
- Hoarseness
- Noisy breathing (stridor)
- Postnasal drip
- Regurgitation
- Weak voice
- Wheezing

Decoding My Problem

For those sufferers who have had previous treatment for GERD, better awareness and new technology have made it easier to make the diagnosis of GERD and LPRD. The newer medicines and combinations of

---

Risk Factors for LPRD

- Alcohol
- Caffeinated beverages
- Eating before bedtime
- Eating foods that are high in fat, high in carbohydrates, tomato-based, or spicy
- Lying down immediately after eating
- Obesity
- Smoking
- Wearing tight clothing

medicines have led to an improvement in overall medical management. Also good dietary direction can now be provided, offering new hope for sufferers. New surgical options are also available when other avenues have been tried, and failed.

Review the results from the GERD/LPRD portion of the CAID Quiz (p. 73). Locate your score so that you can define your next course of action, and follow these guidelines:

- If your score is 0–10, you can treat yourself with over-the-counter (OTC) medicines.
- If your score is 11–25, you need to see your primary-care physician and follow the protocol provided later in this chapter.
- If your score is 26–45, you need to see a gastroenterologist.
- If your score is 46 or more, you need to see an ear, nose, and throat (ENT) doctor who specializes in treating CAID or at least has an understanding of the relationship between sinus disease and GERD/LPRD.

Your Visit with an ENT Specialist

After your ENT doctor takes a detailed medical history, he or she will perform a head and neck examination with a focus on the nose and the throat. If your doctor thinks that you may have LPRD, he or she may perform a throat examination using a small mirror. The doctor may also use an instrument called a flexible fiber-optic laryngoscope. This is a thin, flexible fiber lens that allows the doctor to look at your voice box and throat.

Before the laryngoscope exam, your nose is sprayed with a decongestant mixed with a mild anesthetic, or the two may be given as separate sprays. The otolaryngologist (ENT doctor) will use the laryngoscope to evaluate your nose, throat, and voice box. If the area is swollen, inflamed, and/or red—especially around your voice box—you might have LPRD. Very often, patients who suffer from LPRD show swelling behind the vocal cords at the top of the esophagus, called postglottic swelling. The ENT is also looking for the following features:

- Red, irritated, and/or swollen arytenoids (structures at the back of the vocal cords that make them move) and/or interarytenoid space (the space between the arytenoids)
- Red, irritated larynx (vocal cords)
- Small laryngeal ulcers
- Swelling of the vocal folds
- Granulomas or polyps on the vocal cords or in the larynx
- Evidence of a hiatal-hernia-like secretions coming up from the esophagus
- Significant laryngeal pathology of any type

A second type of examination is called a videostroboscopy. This is a video examination of the larynx using a rigid endoscope with an intermittent (strobe) xenon light source that is activated by vocal fold movement. The video examination allows enlarged, slow-motion visualization of the vocal cords. This technology is also available for use in the doctor's office and begins with a topical spray anesthesia. The definitive diagnosis of LPRD is made by demonstrating that there is acid reflux into the back of the throat. To do this, two pH sensors are used, and the patient is monitored over a 24-hour period. A small tube is passed through the nose into the esophagus to monitor the amount and type of reflux during a typical day. The patient is then free to leave the office, returning the next day. One of the biggest advantages of this type of testing is that it allows the monitoring of the patient's system while he or she goes through a typical daily routine. In some cases, barium studies (X-ray test) are used. This procedure is almost always done if a patient complains of difficulty with swallowing, because it will clearly show if there are any scars or abnormal growths in the esophagus or if there is any inflammation of the esophagus caused by refluxed acid. A study called an esophagealgastroduodenal (EGD) endoscopy can be used to evaluate the esophagus, stomach, and small intestine for related conditions. Although barium esophagoscopy is less sensitive in diagnosing LPRD, it is often used after treatment has failed.

Last, some physicians take a biopsy—either by using a brush to gather cells (called a brush biopsy) or by actually taking a piece of tissue—as a means for identifying changes in the lining of the throat that correspond to chronic irritation due to reflux. Some children have nonacidic reflux, which is not picked up by a pH probe or biopsy, and new studies are under way to determine whether a different type of probe can be used to identify this condition.

Nonmedical Options for Treating LPRD

There are many lifestyle changes that you can make to control or prevent GERD/LPRD. I call this my gastroesophageal (GE) Reflux Recommendations.

GE REFLUX RECOMMENDATIONS

Do not smoke, and if you do quit immediately. Among the many dangers of smoking is that it will cause and exacerbate reflux disease by irritating the membranes of the stomach, esophagus, nose, and sinuses.

Try to maintain a healthy body weight. Being overweight can dramatically increase reflux. Being overweight causes a shift in the position of the GE junction. For patients with recent weight gain, shedding a few pounds is often all that is required to control reflux. You don't have to lose 50 pounds in 1 week. Instead, try to lose ½ pound per week until you lose the desired amount of weight. This is a very realistic goal and can be accomplished by modifying your diet, developing good eating habits, staying well hydrated, and exercising. I tell my patients to eat three to four small meals daily, instead of fewer, larger meals. Don't skip meals, especially breakfast.

Pay close attention to how your system reacts to various foods.
We each have distinct foods that cause an increase in our reflux. The foods
that are most often reactive are caffeine, cola beverages, acidic fruits and
their juices (orange or tomato juice), mints, spicy foods, acidic and
tomato-based foods (Mexican or Italian) alcoholic beverages (particularly
at night), cheese, fried foods, eggs, and chocolate. Carbohydrates, including breads, pasta, and rice, are also thought to cause reflux. By avoiding
these foods entirely, you may see a significant change in your reflux. You
can then add them back into your diet, one food group at a time for 1
week to see what the culprit is.

Stay away from tight belts and restrictive clothing. Weight loss will
also help you avoid tight-fitting clothes that exacerbate reflux problems.
Tight-fitting clothes will also shift the position of your GE junction.

Avoid bedtime snacks. Your last meal should be finished no less
than 3 hours before bedtime. Food left in your stomach before you go
to sleep will reflux into your esophagus. If you give yourself time to
properly digest your food before you go to sleep, the food has time to
pass from the stomach down to the intestines where it will no longer
reflux into the esophagus after you lie down. Therefore, if you feel
like having dessert, eat your ice cream right after dinner, not as you
are sliding into bed. In fact, avoiding eating a large meal at night will
help greatly. Your body will be better able to digest food throughout
the day.

Drink water all day long. You need to stay well hydrated. This will
keep the material in your stomach moving. It will keep your membranes
moist, and replenish the water in all of the cells of your body, keeping
them healthy.

**Make time in your schedule to do activities that lower your
stress level.** Avoid stress and take significant steps to reduce stress. Even
moderate stress can dramatically increase the amount of reflux. It also in-

creases the amount of acids released in your stomach. Decreasing stress will reduce reflux. Try meditation, yoga, or light exercise every day. However, do not exercise immediately after eating because this can shift the position of the GE junction.

Elevate the head of your bed 4–6 inches. This will allow gravity to help decrease reflux that may occur when you are lying flat on your back. You can use books, bricks, or a block of wood under the legs of the head of your bed to achieve a 10- to 15-degree slant. Do not prop up your head and neck with extra pillows. This may increase reflux by kinking the stomach. Recent studies have shown that reflux occurs much more often during the day when upright; therefore, raising your bed may be much less important than once believed.

Gargle with a glass of salt water twice a day before you brush your teeth. You should use ¼ teaspoon of salt in an 8-ounce glass of water. This will soothe the irritation and wash the stomach acid from the membranes.

By following these recommendations, you may be able to skip GERD/LPRD medications entirely.

Lauren, a 58-year-old executive, came to see me because of her chronic coughing. She worked late hours and had to frequently wine and dine her clients. She usually felt fine, but when one of her coughing bouts began, it could go on for days. Lauren told me that she felt as if something were caught in her throat, but nothing she did could alleviate the feeling, even at night. The feeling once was so severe that she was rushed to the hospital; but by the time she got there, the episode had passed.

It is interesting that Lauren did not suffer from sinus problems, heartburn, or indigestion, and she didn't think that she had reflux. She didn't burp, and she was not overweight. She occasionally had late-night snacks before going to bed, and admitted to me that her eating habits were not good. Her breakfast consisted of two quick cups of coffee. She occasionally ate lunch but usually skipped the meal because she knew she would be eating a large dinner out with clients. Dinner was usually accompanied by a few social drinks. During the day, she drank a lot of coffee and soda to keep alert, and she did not feel hungry.

Lauren was seen by her internist and various consultants for her coughing. They all agreed that Lauren was not suffering from sinus problems, and placed her on GERD medications, although nothing relieved her cough. She was diagnosed with panic attacks and had been seeing a psychiatrist who placed her on various medicines, also without results. She was then referred to my office.

Using a fiber-optic nasopharyngolaryngoscope, I was able to make the diagnosis of silent GERD (LPRD). I suggested my GE Reflux Recommendations. Lauren stopped drinking alcohol at dinner, and replaced her caffeine fix with bottled water and lemonade. She started to eat a small breakfast, a medium-size lunch, and cut down on the size of her dinners. She eliminated carbohydrates from most of her meals, and made sure that her last meal was finished at least 3 hours before going to sleep. She now includes exercise as part of her daily routine, which keeps her stress levels down. Within a month Lauren came back and told me that she feels much better. Her coughing has not returned, and she finally has uninterrupted sleep. Best of all, she is no longer taking any medicines.

Medical Options for Treating LPRD

If you have followed the GE Reflux Recommendations and still feel uncomfortable, you might want to consider medications, either OTC or prescription remedies. Because of the distinct relationship between GERD/LPRD and CAID, if you are experiencing symptoms that are associated with sinus disease as well as GERD, you might want to try to treat your sinus symptoms either first, or at least concurrently. Refer to Chapter 5 for treatments for your particular sinus symptoms.

I find that most individuals with LPRD require medication to control their acid reflux. There are three main classes of medications used to treat LPRD:

- Antacids
- H$_2$-blockers
- Proton pump inhibitors (PPIs)

ANTACIDS

Antacids are medications that work by neutralizing acid that is already in the stomach. Antacids usually contain calcium, aluminum, or magnesium. Antacids containing magnesium tend to have a laxative action; those containing aluminum may cause constipation. Magnesium carbonate works by liberating carbon dioxide from the stomach, and can cause frequent belching. Alginates, such as sodium alginate, are another common ingredient of indigestion or heartburn remedies. These work by forming a protective coating over the walls of the stomach and esophagus.

No matter which antacid remedy you choose, it is best to take them after a meal, especially if you drank alcohol with the meal or if you plan to go to sleep less than 3 hours after eating.

OTC Antacids and Ingredients

Gaviscon
Aluminum hydroxide, 95 mg
Magnesium hydroxide, 110 mg

Maalox
Aluminum hydroxide, 200 mg
Magnesium hydroxide, 200 mg
Simethicone, 20 mg

Maalox Max
Aluminum hydroxide, 400 mg
Magnesium hydroxide, 400 mg
Simethicone, 40 mg

Maalox Chewable
Calcium carbonate, 600 mg

Maalox Max Chewable
Calcium carbonate, 1,000 mg
Simethicone, 60 mg

Mylanta
Aluminum hydroxide, 200 mg
Magnesium hydroxide, 200 mg
Simethicone, 20 mg

Mylanta Maximum Strength
Aluminum hydroxide, 400 mg
Magnesium hydroxide, 400 mg
Simethicone, 40 mg

Rolaids
Calcium carbonate, 500 mg
Magnesium hydroxide, 110 mg

Rolaids Multisymptom
Calcium carbonate, 675 mg
Magnesium hydroxide, 135 mg
Simethicone, 60 mg

Titralac
Calcium carbonate, 420 mg

Titralac Plus
Calcium carbonate, 420 mg
Simethicone, 21 mg

Tums
Calcium carbonate, 500 mg

H_2-BLOCKERS

H_2-blockers are drugs that block the histamine receptors in the stomach to reduce acid secretion. The chemical histamine, the same substance released during an allergic reaction, stimulates certain cells in the stomach to produce acid. It does this by attaching, or binding, to a particular site on those cells—known as H_2-receptors. An H_2-antagonist, or blocker, works by binding to H_2-receptors, and thus "blocks" the cells from producing acid.

Because H_2-blockers are used to reduce acid secretion in the stomach, they are not effective once you begin experiencing the symptoms of LPRD. To be effective, they must be taken regularly before meals. H_2-blockers cause relatively few side effects. The most common are diarrhea and other digestive disturbances, headache, dizziness, and tiredness, or hair loss with Tagamet (cimetidine) and sweating with Axid (nizatidine). One H_2-blocker, Zantac (ranitidine, bismuth citrate), can cause the tongue to darken and stools to turn black. H_2-blockers are often prescribed in addition to PPIs. These medications come in OTC and prescription formulas. Some common H_2-blockers are nizatidine (Axid), famotidine (Pepcid), cimetidine (Tagament), and ranitidine (Zantac).

PROTON PUMP INHIBITORS

PPIs are the newest and most effective medications used to treat GERD/LPRD. This class of medicines works by completely blocking the production of stomach acid. They do this by shutting down a system in the stomach known as the "proton pump." They work best when taken 30–60 minutes before eating a meal that contains protein, such as meat, cheese, or fish. If you take the medicine once a day, it is important to take it 30–60 minutes before you eat your largest meal, usually dinner. If you take the medicine twice a day, take one dose 60 minutes before breakfast and one dose 60 minutes before dinner. If you do not eat dinner, take the medicine 60 minutes before lunch.

Proton pump inhibitors generally don't cause many side effects. The most common side effects are diarrhea, a feeling of being sick, constipation, abdominal pain, and headaches. They can also cause allergic reactions, itching, dizziness, swollen ankles, muscle and joint pain, blurred vision, depression, and a dry mouth—although these reactions are rare. These medications come in OTC and prescription formulas. Some common proton pump inhibitors are rabeprazole sodium (AcipHex), esomeprazole magnesium (Nexium), lansoprazole (Prevacid), omeprazole (Prilosec), and pantoprazole sodium (Protonix).

If you are diagnosed with LPRD, the principal therapy will include a PPI. Within 2–3 months of treatment, most people will report a reduction in their symptoms. After 3 months, PPI therapy can be weaned off. However, if symptoms return once off of medication, therapy can be continued indefinitely.

Robert was a 38-year-old man who came to the office complaining of waking up at night and feeling as if he were suffocating. This experience had been going on for 3 months. He had a history of some minor allergies and had sinus problems for years. Robert complained that when his sinuses acted up, he suffered from bad sinus headaches. His wife, Constance, reported that Robert also snored and often woke up with a stiff neck. He had nasal congestion with recurrent infections and yellowish mucus, which passed back into his throat. As a result, he had a chronic cough and frequently found himself clearing his throat to get rid of the mucus. With these coughing fits, his reflux would act up. Constance told me that she could tell when Robert was getting a sinus infection because his breath smelled moldy, like a humid locker room. Furthermore, Constance could also tell when Robert's reflux acted up because his breath got sour. In fact, she was so astute, that she was able to discern which sign was the initial trigger: She could always smell the sinus infection first, and the smell itself became sour as his reflux symptoms become worse and Robert's voice turned hoarse.

A surgeon had told Robert that he needed sinus surgery. I decided to treat Robert with antibiotics and nasal steroid sprays first to clear up his sinus infection. I requested that he follow my GE Reflux Recommendations, and started him with a PPI.

After 3 months, Robert came back to my office. He had lost some weight and reported a considerable improvement. He noted that with the new GERD medication, he felt like a new person. His reflux rarely acted up; and when it did, it was usually when he forgot to take his medicines. Now his sinus infections are very infrequent and remarkably less severe; and when they do occur, a quick course of antibiotics usually clears them up. He likes his nasal spray and is quite compliant with his saline irrigation. Best of all, Robert was able to forego surgery by following the CAID medication regimen and GE Reflux Recommendations.

Surgical Options

I frequently find that my patients with GERD/LPRD often feel relief from their symptoms after sinus surgery. However, if your reflux problem is severe, or the excess acid cannot be controlled by medication, your doctor may recommend gastrointestinal procedures and/or surgery.

Gastroenterologists have been performing different procedures that decrease the gastroesophageal reflux, thereby avoiding surgery. These include endoscopic suturing, radiofrequency ablation, and injection of an inert polymer to bolster the lower esophageal sphincter.

Surgery to treat reflux disease is the last resort and should not be taken lightly. The main objective of surgery is to tighten the junction between the stomach and esophagus so acid does not wash into the esophagus. The surgery most commonly done is called the Nissen fundoplication. This surgery will create a new and better valve between the esophagus and the stomach to prevent the acid from backing into your throat or voice box. For more information about this surgery, consult with a chest surgeon who specializes in this procedure. A general surgeon, gastroenterologist, or thoracic surgeon will perform an evaluation to determine if surgery is necessary.

CHAPTER 8

GETTING A GOOD NIGHT'S SLEEP: COMBATING SNORING AND SLEEP APNEA

Sleep occupies a third of our lives, yet for many of us, sleep is not the pleasant experience it is supposed to be. If you are suffering from chronic airway-digestive inflammatory disease (CAID), you might not be getting a restful sleep because either your nose is congested, and/or you have other blockages in your airway that cause you to snore.

Snoring seems innocuous, but in fact it makes many people miserable. Those who snore can unknowingly be awakened several times during the night and are often tired during the day, even though they might think they slept well. In addition, one person's snoring commonly affects the sleep of their significant other as well as everyone else in the household. You may even have experienced leaving the bedroom in the middle of the night so that your partner can sleep. It's then no surprise that snoring is the number one medical reason for divorce. Approximately 25 percent of Americans snore, with a larger percentage of male snorers, almost four to one. Men begin to snore in their 20s or 30s, whereas women usually don't complain of snoring until their 50s.

Many sufferers of CAID also experience sleep apnea, a serious medical condition that can be fatal. Sleep apnea occurs when snoring is interrupted by silent pauses, during which time the person stops breathing because his or her airway has become completely blocked. The individual's oxygen levels drop: the brain and heart do not get the oxygen that they need. This condition is directly linked to heart disease, heart attack, and stroke. Therefore, if you know that you snore or have been told that you snore, it is important that you not only treat your symptoms but determine whether or not you are suffering from sleep apnea. Unfortunately, because snoring and apnea cause no pain to the sufferer, most people do not seek help, unless their significant other forces them to. Even then, sufferers, to their own detriment, are reluctant about seeking treatment.

What Is Snoring?

Snoring is a noise produced during sleep, occurring when you either inhale or exhale through your nose and mouth at the same time. The noise is made by the palate and the uvula flapping as you breathe. The flapping sensation worsens when the size of the breathing passageway decreases due to obstruction, inflammation, or an anatomical narrowing anywhere from the tip of the nose to the back of the throat. The physics behind breathing calls for the lungs to pull against an exact resistance. That is why when your nose is clogged you assist your nose by breathing through a slight opening of your mouth. At night, as the airway decreases, the lungs need to pull harder to get air in and will have to exhale with increased force to blow the air out. This increase in pressure causes the palate and uvula to flap, leading to the sound of snoring. This can sound like a soft purr or like someone is sawing wood.

Often, the muscles associated with the structures at the back of the throat relax, causing the airway to collapse, thereby worsening the vibration in the soft palate, uvula, or sometimes the tonsils. This collapse can occur when there is either extra tissue in the back of the airway (such as when you have enlarged tonsils), a decrease in the tone of the muscles holding the airway open, or if the tongue is so relaxed it falls back and closes off the airway. While the snoring noise does not come from the nose itself, but from the palate, people with nasal obstruction due to sinusitis, nasal anatomical narrowing, or allergies typically snore more than those who do not suffer from CAID.

Many physicians will argue that sinus or nasal obstruction does not lead to snoring or sleep apnea. I have found that this is not the case: there is a direct link between the two conditions. For many, their nasal valve can be structurally too narrow or easily collapsible; and when this area is opened up with either a mechanical device or surgery, these patients find that their snoring disappears or improves. Typically, the worse the nasal and sinus obstruction, the louder the snoring. Furthermore, the position of your tongue is another important contributing factor.

Snoring and Your Weight

Snoring can also be caused by weight gain. When you put on a few extra pounds, you may notice it in your face, belly, and legs, but your size is also increasing in places that are less obvious, including your nose, throat, and tongue. As you gain weight, you are also building layers of fat around the airway, decreasing its diameter. Any small change in your airway will greatly reduce its surface area. This causes your lungs to pull hard during inhalation and push hard during exhalation to get air through, which again causes your palate to vibrate, leading to the noise of snoring.

People who suffer from snoring can also be overweight, as defined by their body mass index (BMI). This is a standard measurement that determines what your optimal body weight range should be. Many people who snore and sleep less than 7 hours per night have high BMIs, and are more likely to be obese than those who sleep peacefully through the night and do not complain of snoring or sleep apnea.

Snoring Remedies

The good news is that you do not have to snore. Snoring can be completely controlled. There are many easy-to-follow solutions so that you and your entire family will sleep better. The options range from the least invasive lifestyle changes to surgery. I would recommend that you work down the ladder until your snoring is remedied. What's more, if you properly treat your CAID symptoms, you may find that your snoring will go away on its own.

ARE YOU OVERWEIGHT?

The first course of action is almost always centered on weight loss. You will need to determine if your weight falls within a healthy range for your BMI. You don't have to look or feel overweight in order for your BMI to be unhealthy. Table 1 has already done the math for you. To use the table, find your height in inches in the left-hand column. Move across the row to find your weight. The number at the top of the column is the BMI for your height and weight. Your BMI is then assessed by categories, according to the National Institutes of Health:

- Underweight = < 18.5
- Normal weight = 18.5–24.9
- Overweight = 25–29.9
- Obese ≥ 30

If your BMI is high, see your primary-care physician. He or she may want to perform a quick blood test to see if your thyroid hormone levels are in order. If your thyroid is underactive, it could be a cause of your weight gain. You can be prescribed a thyroid hormone treatment that will control your gland: This simple step might lead to immediate

| TABLE 1. BODY MASS INDEX | | | | | | | | | | | | | |
BMI (KG/M^2)	19	20	21	22	23	24	25	26	27	28	29	30	35	40
Height (in.)	Weight (lb.)													
58	91	96	100	105	110	115	119	124	129	134	138	143	167	191
59	94	99	104	109	114	119	124	128	133	138	143	148	173	198
60	97	102	107	112	118	123	128	133	138	143	148	153	179	204
61	100	106	111	116	122	127	132	137	143	148	153	158	185	211
62	104	109	115	120	126	131	136	142	147	153	158	164	191	218
63	107	113	118	124	130	135	141	146	152	158	163	169	197	225
64	110	116	122	128	134	140	145	151	157	163	169	174	204	232
65	114	120	126	132	138	144	150	156	162	168	174	180	210	240
66	118	124	130	136	142	148	155	161	167	173	179	186	216	247
67	121	127	134	140	146	153	159	166	172	178	185	191	223	255
68	125	131	138	144	151	158	164	171	177	184	190	197	230	262
69	128	135	142	149	155	162	169	176	182	189	196	203	236	270
70	132	139	146	153	160	167	174	181	188	195	202	207	243	278
71	136	143	150	157	165	172	179	186	193	200	208	215	250	286
72	140	147	154	162	169	177	184	191	199	206	213	221	258	294
73	144	151	159	166	174	182	189	197	204	212	219	227	265	302
74	148	155	163	171	179	186	194	202	210	218	225	233	272	311
75	152	160	168	176	184	192	200	208	216	224	232	240	279	319
76	156	164	172	180	189	197	205	213	221	230	238	246	287	328

Source: Evidence Report of Clinical Guidelines on the Identification, Evaluation, and Treatment of Overweight and Obesity in Adults, 1998. National Institutes of Heatlh/National Heart, Lung, and Blood Institute (NIH/NHLBI).

weight loss. It is important for you to treat your thyroid because weight gain is only one of the problems that you may encounter from having a low level of thyroid hormone.

I also check my patients to make sure that they are not anemic (low red blood cell levels). Anemia prevents the body from losing weight and can cause fluid retention. Additional iron supplements are necessary for better cell function and metabolism, and the primary reason for the anemia also needs to be uncovered. When an anemia workup is necessary, I typically work closely with the primary-care physician and, if needed, an endocrinologist or a hematologist so that we can treat the anemia appropriately.

If your thyroid is working properly and you are not anemic, you'll need to begin a weight-loss regimen. If you have more than 30 pounds to lose to reach a normal BMI, you might consult a nutritionist, primary-care physician, osteopath, or chiropractor who can develop a diet specific to your needs. Of course, a daily exercise routine is also helpful for weight loss.

An eating regimen that leads to weight loss and curbs snoring would primarily consist of a low-fat, high-protein diet, steering away from carbohydrates, especially at night. Carbohydrates do not directly affect snoring but metabolize into excess fat cells: The carbohydrate molecules that are not burned during the day will convert into body fat in a very short period of time. Alcohol adds lots of empty calories. All alcoholic beverages contain substantial calories and some alcohols are a form of carbohydrate. As a result, alcohol should be avoided; it can cause a flare-up of CAID, the extra calories lead to weight gain, and its sedative effect causes muscle flaccidity and collapse of the airway—all further aggravating the conditions that produce snoring.

Those who are dieting should eat three to four small meals a day, instead of skipping meals and eating larger portions. Frequent, smaller meals help keep your metabolism burning at a higher rate, thereby burning more calories. The last meal of the day should be eaten at least 3 hours before going to sleep. Many people do not eat breakfast or skip lunch, and then have a large dinner and go straight to sleep. This is not good: By following this eating schedule, you are not giving your body enough waking hours to digest such a heavy meal. A large meal and a couple of alcoholic drinks before you go to bed is a recipe for disaster for both your overall health and specifically for your snoring. What's more, eating one meal a day slows down your metabolism and causes you to gain weight. Some people report that if they eat a larger lunch and a smaller dinner, their snoring significantly improves.

In addition, you should drink plenty of water—going to the bathroom a few times a day and having clear urine. Staying well hydrated is good for your entire body, including your skin, heart, circulatory, respiratory, and gastrointestinal (GI) tract. If you eat right, stay well hydrated, and exercise, you will start to lose weight.

My patient Evan is a 51-year-old senior executive who came in complaining of a sinus infection. When asked if he snored, Evan became embarrassed. His wife, Laura, who was sitting with us in the examining room looked up toward the ceiling and started to laugh. "Are you kidding?" she said. "I haven't slept well in years!" I reassured Evan that snoring was common and that there was nothing to be ashamed about.

Just by looking at him, I could tell that Evan needed to lose a few pounds. A BMI table showed that he needed to lose about 15 pounds to reach the top of the normal range, but he could probably stand to lose another 10 pounds as well. I found that Evan had an acute sinus infection, causing him significant nasal obstruction, which was also contributing to his snoring.

I started Evan's treatment with an antibiotic to clear up his sinus infection and placed him on a nasal steroid spray, which brought down some of his nasal swelling. I told him about his need to lose weight and arranged for him to meet with a nutritionist. I also told him to follow Dr. Gary Josephson's (my brother's) protocol for hydration: Every morning Evan was to fill a large thermos with ice and sliced lemons or lime and top it off with water. He was told to keep the thermos at his desk and drink from it throughout the day, filling it back up when the water was gone. This would force him to drink at least 2–3 liters of fluids daily. We made another appointment for him to come back in 6 weeks so I could check on his progress.

When Evan came back, he was proud to share with me that he had lost more than 10 pounds, and his wife reported that his snoring had significantly improved. Evan had started to exercise and eat right, and he was staying well hydrated. Over the next 5 months, Evan lost a total of 21 pounds. Even Laura is now sleeping soundly, and Evan is much happier not sleeping on the couch.

If you follow the tips I gave Evan for an entire month and don't see any results, I strongly suggest that you continue to diet while under the care of a physician and a nutritionist, or other health-care provider. I do not recommend taking over-the-counter (OTC) or prescription diet pills unless you are under the care of a physician.

Lifestyle Changes

While you are working toward losing weight—or if weight loss has been achieved or deemed unnecessary—and you continue to snore, the second set of treatments are habitual or lifestyle changes. First, I always recommend to my patients who snore that they change their body position at night. I find that most people who snore sleep on their backs: Snoring decreases significantly when you sleep on your side and almost goes away entirely if you can learn to sleep on your stomach. By making this simple change, you'll find that your snoring may improve dramatically.

There have been various contraptions sold over the years that will gently remind you to get off your back. You can also try to kick this habit by wearing a pocket T-shirt or dress shirt to bed with the breast pocket on your back. Place a tennis ball in the pocket, and lie down on your side. During the night, if you roll over on your back, you'll instantly feel the ball, making it uncomfortable to sleep on your back, and you will shift your position to either your side or your stomach.

Appliances and Dilators

If you have a history of nasal obstruction stemming from any of the branches of CAID, you can try this low-cost solution: a nasal dilator. These breathing strips are sold over the counter and do not require a prescription. The strip is placed on the outside of the nose, helping the narrowest part of the airway dilate. The breathing strips create a tent, widening the nasal valve, thereby opening the nostrils and the nasal valve area so that the air passage is widened. There are also other types of nasal dilators that are inserted into the nostrils that achieve the same effect.

Oral sleeping devices can also be helpful. These appliances move the lower jaw forward, thereby moving the tongue forward, and keeping it away from the airway. As a result, palate vibration will decrease or disappear. Some custom-made oral appliances fit around your teeth, like a mouth guard. This piece can either be made by an oral surgeon or a dentist specializing in prosthetics of this type. These mouth guards are similar to temporomandibular joint (TMJ) devices. As a result, this may also help you stop grinding your teeth, relieving painful nighttime headaches from TMJ.

Other appliances include a chin strap: an elastic strap that goes around the head and chin, forcing the mouth to stay in the correct position and reducing the loudness of snoring. A removable nasal stent can also be placed inside the nose to open the airway down to the throat. The stent is inserted just before you go to bed.

Any of these tools can provide some relief, depending on your particular case. Unfortunately these appliances cannot cure your snoring problem; they can only place you in a better position so that you do not snore. It's also important to remember that for any of these appliances to work, you must use them faithfully. As soon as you stop, you will begin to snore again.

Aside from these tools, I also recommend using nasal irrigation just before going to bed. You can use a spray bottle, a neti pot or a nasal irrigator, as outlined in Chapter 4. I also recommend breathing steam from a humidifier or vaporizer, or taking a long shower before you go to sleep. All of these techniques will keep the nasal passageways moist and clean.

Last, if you find that your congestion is worse at night, sleeping on two or more pillows, or raising the head of your bed by placing blocks under the legs can be helpful in decreasing the swelling in your nose associated with lying down.

Medications

If you have difficulty breathing through your nose during the day, your CAID treatment may improve your nighttime snoring. However, if you can breathe comfortably during the day, and your only problem is at night when you are lying down, then you may have a borderline nasal obstruction that worsens with lying down. Either of these problems can be treated with medications, either prescription or OTC. Occasionally, you can take a low dosage of oral decongestants if you are acutely congested, often as small as a pediatric dose. Don't forget that decongestants are like amphetamines and can affect your heart and prostate over the long term. Thus I do not recommend long courses of oral decongestants and rarely recommend topical nasal decongestants. Instead, I often prescribe nasal steroid sprays, which are great at reducing the inflammation that can cause snoring.

Surgery

If your snoring does not resolve with simple measures, I recommend that you speak with an ear, nose, and throat (ENT) physician who specializes in snoring. More drastic cases may require surgery, which will enlarge and stabilize the airway by stiffening the palate. Some forms of surgery can be performed in the doctor's office under local anesthesia.

Snore plasty injections are one of the easiest forms of treatment. This procedure is done by injecting an agent into the back of the soft palate that creates a small scar, which helps reduce the vibrations. You may require multiple injections over the course of this treatment: each one lasts between 3 months and 1 year. A second procedure, known as somnoplasty, involves using radiofrequency to cause scarring in the palatal muscle to stiffen the palate. Another new procedure involves inserting three tiny implants, made of woven polyester material, into the palate muscle structure. This operation, known as the pillar procedure, also stiffens the soft palate. Finally, a laser-assisted uvulopalatoplasty (LAUP) can be performed. This procedure tends to be a bit more painful. During this procedure, the surgeon numbs your throat and uses a laser to make cuts into the palate and at the same time shortens and/or removes the uvula. Each of these surgeries claims to have a success rate of close to 90 percent. However, your surgeon must figure out exactly where the problem is to understand which procedure is right for you. They all seem to be effective, although some ENTs are more familiar with one procedure than another. It's best to choose a physician you are comfortable with, and see which technique he or she prefers.

Sinus and nasal surgery may also resolve your snoring. While there is no specific sinus surgery that treats snoring directly, any improvement made to your nasal air flow will positively affect your nighttime breathing and improve your overall sleep.

Andre was more than willing to share his snoring story. Andre was a 45-year-old oral surgeon who came to see me about his snoring. He suffered from chronic sinusitis and a septal deviation and had surgery for his problems. Yet he still continued to snore so loudly that he woke up everyone in the house. I decided to do a pillar procedure. Within one week of the surgery, Andre was pleased to report that he no longer snored, and his entire family is sleeping more peacefully.

Sleep Apnea

Some habitual snorers feel incredibly fatigued, and often find themselves falling asleep during the day. They may unwittingly fall asleep during even the shortest car rides, while watching a movie, or even during business meetings. These same people may have difficulty falling asleep at night or wake up repeatedly to go to the bathroom.

If you are experiencing these symptoms, you might have sleep apnea, a potentially dangerous condition that needs to be treated. *Apnea* means the "absence of breathing," and *sleep apnea* is defined as "a stoppage of breathing for 10 seconds or more while asleep." As many as 4 in 100 men and 2 in 100 women have sleep apnea. Most people are affected as they get older, but I also see young men and women—as well as children—who suffer from this problem.

Nighttime breathing can stop when people who snore or suffer from CAID have episodes of upper-airway obstruction to the point at which the airway is completely blocked for a short period of time.

When this happens, the airway cannot supply oxygen to the body. Instead, those with sleep apnea must rely on their brains to make sure that they continue to breathe. Even in the deepest stages of the sleep cycle, their brain must remind them to wake up and take a deep breath. Often, this reminder is less than gentle: It must be with such a force that it causes a sudden alertness, often in the form of loud snorts or gasps that literally wake up the sufferer and his or her sleeping partner. And because these people are constantly waking up throughout the night, they are not getting refreshing sleep.

OBSTRUCTIVE SLEEP APNEA

Sleep apnea is caused by two distinct problems. In the first rare form, the brain does not relay the message to breathe. This is called central apnea and is caused by an excessive loss of muscle tone following a neurological problem in the brain. This form of sleep apnea is related to narcolepsy (an extreme condition of excessive daytime sleepiness coupled with the sudden loss of voluntary muscle tone, vivid hallucinations during sleep, or brief episodes of total paralysis at the beginning or end of sleep).

The second, more common form is called obstructive sleep apnea (OSA). Like snoring, OSA is caused by an obstruction in the airway, anywhere from the tip of the nose to the back of the throat, including a septal deviation, sinus inflammation, nasal polyps, enlarged tonsils, an enlarged base of tongue, and/or a floppy palate. Those with OSA may be deprived of oxygen for as much as one third of their night's sleep. However, the effects of OSA are mainly felt during the waking hours, when patients are fatigued.

OSA is a chronic progressive disorder that cannot be cured but can be effectively treated. In the United States alone, nearly 30 million people are affected by OSA. Yet, only 8–10 percent of OSA sufferers have been diagnosed and treated. OSA affects approximately 5 percent of men over 50, which is as common as adult asthma. OSA is often misdiagnosed as either attention deficit disorder (ADD) or chronic fatigue syndrome and is one of the leading causes of work- and driving-related accidents. Children can also suffer from OSA, and I believe that many children diagnosed as ADD really suffer from OSA. These children can be cranky; perform poorly in school; and experience night walking, loud snoring, and bedwetting.

You might be inclined to forego treatment for your sleep apnea, and learn to live with your fatigue. However, this line of thinking is dangerous for any aspect of CAID and especially for sleep apnea. Sleep apnea puts an incredible strain on the heart and lungs. Studies have suggested that the OSA syndrome may be an important risk factor for high blood pressure, heart attack, and stroke. In a groundbreaking study, it was revealed that an increased severity of sleep apnea was associated with an increased risk of the development of stroke or death from any cause, meaning that it has a compounding property in relation to age, sex, weight, stress, and other recognizable risk factors. Furthermore, there are strong comorbidity correlations between OSA and hypertension (40–50 percent), congestive heart failure (34 percent), pulmonary disease (11 percent), coronary artery disease (34 percent), fibromyalgia (80 percent), diabetes (65 percent), end-stage kidney disease (50 percent), and even erectile dysfunction (50 percent).

THE SIGNS AND SYMPTOMS OF OSA

If you or someone you know suffers from CAID, snores regularly, and has one or more of the following symptoms, it may be OSA. Symptoms will get worse with age and weight gain:

- Chronic snoring, interrupted by pauses in breathing
- Depression
- Excessive sleepiness or fatigue during the day
- Frequent nighttime urination
- Gasping or choking during sleep
- High blood pressure
- Irritability
- Memory loss
- Migraine headaches
- Morning headache
- Poor judgment or concentration
- Prostate problems
- Restless sleep
- Sexual dysfunction
- Uncontrolled diabetes

GERD AND SLEEP APNEA

Gastroesophageal reflux disease (GERD) may also be connected to sleep apnea. In an important study by the American College of Gastroenterology, it was found that patients with sleep complaints, but without heartburn symptoms, still suffered episodes of nighttime acid reflux. In a separate study, researchers found that symptoms of GERD are common and frequently severe in people with obstructive sleep apnea.

People with gastroesophageal reflux commonly report poor sleep and waking at night because of acid reflux. However, one study showed that 94 percent of the recorded reflux events were associated with arousal from sleep or awakening whether or not the people noticed their reflux. This silent reflux may be the cause of sleep disturbances in people with unexplained sleep disorders. In another study on GERD and sleep presented by researchers at Duke University Medical Center, reflux symptoms were common and frequently severe in 168 patients undergoing sleep studies who reported symptoms consistent with sleep apnea. Therefore, I believe that GERD may be an underlying cause of sleep apnea and needs to be treated appropriately to resolve the sleep apnea.

Diagnosing Sleep Apnea

Luckily, sleep apnea is both easily identified and effectively treated. The most important first step is to keep a sleep diary for 2 weeks. The sleep diary will help your doctor determine your sleeping patterns. Every morning, write down what time you went to bed, what time you got up, how many times you awoke during the night, and if you felt rested when you woke up. At the end of the day, note if you took any naps during the day.

With your sleep diary in hand, speak with your primary-care physician. Your doctor will want to know your symptoms and how long you have had them. If you have a spouse or partner, bring him or her with you to your initial consultation. Snoring and sleep apnea are conditions few want to admit, and most of the time they are not recognized by the sufferer because they don't remember having episodes. Frequently, the best description of a problem will come from someone living with the sufferer.

PARTICIPATING IN A SLEEP STUDY

If your doctor believes that you have sleep apnea, he or she will suggest that you participate in an overnight sleep study, also known as a polysomnogram. The polysomnogram is the only accurate way to determine your condition. It charts your brain waves, heart beat, arm and leg movement, and breathing patterns as you sleep.

You will not feel any pain during the polysomnogram. During a sleep study, sensors are placed on your head, face, chest, and legs, which send signals to a computer that records when you are asleep and awake during the night. The wires are long enough to let you move around and turn over in bed. Breathing monitors show the number of times you stop breathing and can detect changes in air flow and disruptions in your blood oxygen level. The leg, eyelid, and chin sensors record both minor twitches and major movements that occur during the night. A clip will also be placed on your finger to note changes in the level of oxygen in your blood. When you are asleep, a low-light videocamera allows a technologist to see you from a nearby room.

A sleep study can also be performed at home. As you can imagine, it is more comfortable to take the sleep study at home and often the results are more quickly determined. At home, you can also do a multiple night study, and avoid night to night variations. Some people sleep well one night and terribly the next, depending on how tired they are and what they ate or drank for dinner.

There are major benefits of home OSA testing units:

- The newest units provide the same sophistication of data collection that overnight testing provides, including sleep staging and a complete sleep profile.
- Units are lightweight, portable, and easy to transport.
- There is a high degree of data integrity and security to ensure accurate test results.

- Wireless and disposable sensors can be easily attached to the body.
- It costs much less than overnight testing.

Treatment for Sleep Apnea

CPAP

If you are diagnosed with OSA, the most common treatment is a continuous positive airway pressure (CPAP) machine. The CPAP machine is no more than a generator connecting a hose to a mask, which you wear to sleep. The treatment works as air is forced out of the generator into the nose and down the lungs. CPAP provides a gentle flow of positive pressure air into your airway to create a larger opening during sleep, thereby circumventing any obstruction.

There is some mild discomfort associated with the machine, and not everyone is able to tolerate the treatment. The CPAP machine is somewhat noisy, which might be troublesome for either the snorer or their partner. Often, wearing the mask causes mild claustrophobia, a dry nose, and the feeling that you can't breathe. Compliance with CPAP is usually horrible, and many of my patients cannot tolerate it at all. However, the change in just one night is so dramatic that it is worth using.

The CPAP machine itself will not cure sleep apnea. However, if you are on a weight-loss program or go for any of the forms of surgery that relieve obstruction, your apnea may be cured, and you may no longer require the CPAP machine. However, until the time that your apnea is cured, use of the machine will allow you a more restful, and safer, night of sleep.

MEDICAL TREATMENTS FOR SLEEP APNEA

Like snoring, OSA is linked to increased weight gain, and there are several medications that can help bring your weight, and therefore your sleep apnea, under control. The medical therapies we previously discussed can open up your airway, possibly relieving your sleep apnea as well. If you are experiencing constant fatigue, lack of motivation, or difficulty concentrating, you may be suffering from excessive sleepiness brought on by sleep apnea. Provigil (modafinil) is a new medication that is often prescribed to improve wakefulness in patients with OSA. Unlike other stimulants such as amphetamines, Provigil is not addictive and will not affect your ability to fall asleep.

SURGICAL TREATMENTS FOR SLEEP APNEA

There are various forms of surgery to treat sleep apnea. Of the treatments that have been mentioned for snoring, the Pillar procedure can also improve mild to moderate sleep apnea. If this does not work, you may want to try the LAUP procedure. Some physicians will perform the LAUP procedure for sleep apnea without even trying the Pillar procedure. However, the LAUP procedure is more invasive and painful. If a LAUP does not work, you may want to contemplate a uvulopalato-plasty procedure (UPPP). A UPPP is performed under general anesthesia: Your tonsils are removed and the palate is shortened. In some patients, especially children, just removing the tonsils and/or adenoids may resolve the snoring and/or sleep apnea.

Other sleep apnea procedures involve changing the anatomy of the tongue and the throat, limiting obstruction. These include a tongue suspension, geniohyoid advancement, and a hyoid suspension. These procedures are usually reserved for severe sleep apnea patients who have failed UPPP and are unable to use the CPAP machine. There are also some orthognathic options that advance the jaw if there is a deformity of the mandible causing your airway to collapse. The decision to perform any these operations is complex and should be discussed with your surgeon.

PART THREE

COMPLETING SINUS RELIEF

CHAPTER 9

SPECIAL-NEEDS PATIENTS

There are two distinct issues for those who suffer from sinus disease as well as other chronic illnesses. First, you need to know if your seemingly unrelated chronic illness is actually causing your chronic airway-digestive inflammatory disease (CAID). Second, you need to know if the treatments you are following for your chronic illness are compatible with the treatments and remedies for CAID. For instance, people with immune disorders (such as systemic lupus), with immunologic deficiencies (including AIDS), or who are taking immunosuppressants as a form of cancer treatment all have special needs regarding sinus disease.

Many different disease processes can cause CAID, including immunologically based disorders. As we discussed in Chapter 1, the sinuses are intimately involved in controlling the body's immune functioning. The mucus that the sinuses secrete is rich in various chemicals and enzymes as well as immunoglobulins. Different diseases, and the medications used to treat them, may impair the body's immune system or decrease its ability to secrete this mucus with normal immunologic function, leading to sinus dysfunction. These disorders, including diabetes, can predispose people to sinus infections.

Syndromes Related to CAID

These sections discuss special situations that stem from CAID symptoms and/or their treatment, and as they relate to various other disorders.

NASAL POLYPS

CAID itself can cause an anatomical change to the interior of the nose. I frequently see patients who have developed nasal polyps; benign tumors that occur when chronic inflammation causes the membranes of the sinuses and nose to swell and form individual or multiple polyps. Nasal polyps can be as small as the tip of a ballpoint pen or as large as a grape. Even small polyps can obstruct sinus openings, which can further aggravate sinusitis. It is one of the worst forms of chronic sinusitis and often occurs when there are issues relating to asthma, allergies, and—in the most aggressive variant—allergy to aspirin.

Polyps can be diagnosed with a computed tomography (CT) scan or by nasal endoscopy, an office procedure in which your ear, nose, and throat (ENT) physician will either place a rigid or a flexible lighted tube (endoscope) into your nose to examine the nasal and sinus passages. To reduce the size of nasal polyps so that breathing can return to normal, you must break the inflammatory cycle. As mentioned, polyps are caused by inflammation, which is caused by infection. I often prescribe nasal steroid sprays or oral steroids, such as prednisone, to reduce inflammation. Topical steroids via irrigation or nebulizer can be a beneficial treatment as well. Antibiotics and/or oral or topical antifungal drugs can also help eliminate any underlying infection. If you have allergies, antihistamines may be required as well.

Polyps may need to be surgically removed if drugs don't help. This outpatient procedure can be performed with local anesthesia, and is discussed further in Chapter 12. What's more, polyps tend to recur, so medication must be continued even after surgery to control them. When they start to grow back, your physician should remove them along with any related infection. I recommend to all of my patients with polyp disease to irrigate daily and use various medicines on a consistent basis.

SAMTER'S TRIAD

Although Samter's triad is rare, when it is present it can be insidious. This syndrome includes chronic sinusitis with nasal polyposis, asthma, and aspirin allergy. This syndrome can look different in each case, because it presents with a disparate set of symptoms. These sufferers usually complain of nasal congestion, lack of sense of smell and taste, yellow-green discharge, postnasal drip, mouth breathing, a drowned or hoarse voice, chapped lips, and mild headaches and/or pressure. They are prone to nasal polyps and their asthma is usually aggressive. Upon further inquiry or testing, allergy to aspirin or other nonsteroidal anti-inflammatory agents, such as ibuprofen, will be discovered.

Samter's triad often occurs in midlife (20s and 30s are the most common onset times) and may or may not include any environmental allergies. Sampter's triad is also known as aspirin-sensitive asthma, aspirin-induced asthma, aspirin triad, or Widal's triad—and to the fully uninformed, as rhinitis. Sampter's patients typically seek medical attention for wheezing or chest tightness (asthma), then polyp formation is discovered, and aspirin sensitivity is revealed. The aspirin reaction can be mild, including a rash or hives and swelling, or it can be severe, including an asthma attack and/or anaphylaxis The exact cause of Samter's triad is unknown, but it is widely believed that the disorder is caused by a genetic abnormality that effects the body's inflammatory response. Treatment typically focuses on each of the symptoms, and includes nasal steroids, inhaled steroids, and leukotriene antagonists. The chronic sinusitis is treated with various medicines such as antibiotics and antifungal medicines as well as irrigation. Surgery may be required to open up obstructed areas of the sinuses and to remove polyps. Typically, the polyps will recur and so it is important for these patients to be under close supervision by a surgeon. The surgeon periodically checks if the polyps have returned. When polyp disease recurs the polyps should be removed immediately to prevent obstruction of the sinus pathways. The infection should be removed as well. Furthermore, these sufferers need to abstain from taking any aspirin or nonsteroidal anti-inflammatory agents. Some people require oral steroids to alleviate asthma and congestion, and most patients will have recurring or chronic sinusitis caused by the nasal inflammation. Leukotriene antagonists and inhibitors such as Singulair, Accolate, and Zyflo show great promise in treating these patients. Frequent irrigation and cleaning with emollients is also recommended to keep the nasal membranes from becoming inflamed, thereby thwarting the growth of polyps before they begin.

KARTAGENER'S SYNDROME

Kartagener's syndrome is a hereditary syndrome. It is characterized by recurrent upper- and lower-respiratory tract infections due to abnormal ciliary structure and function. This disease is also known as immotile cilia syndrome. Its main characteristic is that the ciliated hair cells on the mucous membranes have impaired movement and therefore can not clear the mucus in the sinuses. Patients with Kartagener's syndrome also suffer from bronchiectasis, chronic sinusitis, situs inversus (the organs are situated on the opposite side from where they are supposed to be), and sterility (because of immotile sperm).

If you have Kartagener's syndrome, you may have experienced chronic, thick, mucus production and an impaired sense of smell since early childhood. Nasal polyps occur in 30 percent of affected individuals. The recurrent chronic sinusitis typically produces sinus pressure headaches over the frontal or maxillary sinuses and around the eyes. You may experience several sinus infections a year that improve with antibiotic therapy but continue to recur.

Treatment is aimed at reducing symptoms and slowing disease progression. This includes antibiotics, steroid nasal sprays, and frequent nasal irrigation.

SARCOIDOSIS

Sarcoidosis is a multisystem inflammatory disorder in which the body forms noncaseating granulomas—benign masses that form in the lungs, sinuses, nose, skin, and occasionally the parotid glands. This disorder commonly affects young adults. Thorough examination of the body on a systemic level is critical to determine if the disease has spread to other organ systems. For example, sarcoidosis may be found in the salivary glands, lymph nodes of the neck, the chest cavity, and lung cavity. It may even be present in the abdominal cavity or retroperitoneal organs (such as the adrenal glands and kidneys) and can cause lesions in the skin.

Sarcoidosis can act up at any time or it can disappear spontaneously. When sarcoidosis flares, you may feel severely fatigued and be inaccurately diagnosed as anemic (low blood count), because of the fatigue. Sarcoidosis is often associated with joint pain, as are many other inflammatory disorders. CAID-related complaints include epistaxis, nasal pain and obstruction, lack of a sense of smell, and hoarseness. It can also affect the nervous system.

Specific blood test results for sarcoidosis might include an elevated sedimentation rate as well as an elevated angiotensin-converting enzyme titer. There often appears to be an imbalance in B and T lymphocyte activity. Chest X-rays and biopsies of the granulomas are the most critical tests for establishing a diagnosis. Once a firm diagnosis is established, an ENT can deal with specific issues such as crusting, bleeding, obstruction of the nasal cavity, and chronic sinus infection caused by blockage of the sinus cavities by these granulomas. While it sometimes requires surgery, it will often require steroids to decrease the inflammation and control the immune system. A good pulmonologist or rheumatologist is critical to directing long-term medical treatment.

SCUBA DIVERS AND FREQUENT FLYERS

I treat many patients with ear and sinus problems resulting from either scuba diving (or snorkeling, or just plain diving into the water) or frequent air travel. Changes in altitude or changes in the depth of the water that you reach are tied to changes in the pressures that your body experiences. With these changes, all of the cavities in your body need to equalize with the outside pressure. However, when any cavity in your body is closed, such as a sinus cavity, or the middle ear (when a eustachian tube is closed) or even a tooth with a filling (if a small air bubble is inadvertently trapped), this equalization may not take place. As a result, there is an abnormal pressure gradient that can cause tearing of the membranes. In the sinuses, this can cause mild to excruciating pressure or pain called sinus squeeze. In the ear, it can cause ear squeeze. This can feel as if someone were stabbing you in these locations. The torn nasal membranes can lead to nosebleeds. When it occurs in the ear, you can end up with temporary or permanent hearing loss, ringing in the ears (tinnitus), or vertigo (dizziness).

Divers and frequent flyers know to equalize their sinuses and ear cavities by swallowing, chewing, or opening the mouth (yes, you can do this under water), or by squeezing the nose and blowing, causing an opening of the sinus cavity or the eustachian tube. It is important for divers and flyers to make sure that their sinuses are working properly so that they can continue to equalize their ear and sinus pressures. When patients have sinus problems, often an eustachian tube is swollen and can cause ear problems.

In addition, even if you have minor inflammation when you start out, both flying and diving can worsen the swelling and cause closure of the sinus cavities and eustachian tubes. When you are on a plane, you are exposed to very dry air, which contains bacteria, viruses, and/or fungi circulating on the plane. Your sinuses may become infected and inflamed, causing swelling and possibly closure, preventing you from equalizing. When the inflammation causes swelling of the eustachian tubes, you may develop problems equalizing your ears. And when the cabin pressure changes, you can develop terrible ear pressure and pain, and/or sinus pressure and pain. For these instances, I have developed quick-and-easy tips to make your flying and diving experiences much more pleasant.

1. Stay well hydrated. Drink plenty of water for at least 1 day before diving or flying.
2. Do not drink alcohol, smoke, or take nonprescription drugs before or around the time of diving or flying.
3. Use plenty of nasal saline spray before and after flying and before diving. You can even bring it on the plane and use it during the flight.

4. Find a method that allows you to open up your eustachian tubes and continue to use it while you are changing altitude. Some methods are swallowing, opening your mouth and moving your jaw around, and (when flying, not diving) chewing gum.

5. Try equalizing your ears by the Valsalva maneuver. The Valsalva maneuver is done by pinching the tip of your nose to close your nostrils, preventing air from escaping. Then blow air into your nose but don't let the air out of your nostrils, thereby forcing the air to open up your sinus passageways and your eustachian tubes. This should lead to a popping of your ears—thus equalizing the pressure. In diving language, this is called clearing your ears.

6. Some flyers and divers take an oral decongestant and others use a nasal decongestant spray before their excursion. This can work, but I caution that these products can also dehydrate you, negating some of the effect. Furthermore, they may interact with your heart, raising your blood pressure and heart rate, which may not be such a good idea, especially before diving. Certainly people with heart disease should refrain from using these decongestants.

If you chronically need to take decongestants before diving or flying, I suggest that you consult with an otolaryngologist (ENT specialist) who understands these particular issues. Preferably, you should find a physician who dives. The Divers Alert Network (DAN) is a nonprofit medical and research organization associated with the Duke University Medical Center that is dedicated to the safety and health of recreational scuba divers. It operates the only 24-hour diving emergency hotline. DAN also operates a diving medical information hotline that can help you find a medical professional in your area who is familiar with diving. These physicians should also understand your problem. Contact DAN through their website (www.diversalertnetwork.org).

The warning signs that tell you that you need to seek help and should not fly or dive before seeing your ENT physician include:

- A recent sinus or ear infection leading to congestion of your nose, sinuses and/or ears, preventing you from clearing your ears

- Difficulty equalizing pressure in your sinuses or ears when in an elevator
- Problems popping your ears with the Valsalva maneuver

WEGENER'S GRANULOMATOSIS

Wegener's granulomatosis affects the respiratory tract from the nose and sinuses to the lungs. It also affects the kidneys. This disease is a systemic inflammatory disease whereby the body creates autoantibodies: antibodies that attack your own organs and body structures. In the nose, sinuses, and face this can lead to a collapse of the sinus structures and your nose. Patients with this disorder also have recurrent sinus infections. One of the primary symptoms is thick crusting with infection in the nasal passageway. Patients might also complain of a foul smell, bleeding, pus, and hard rock-like crusts. These patients can also experience swelling of their salivary glands, but this is rare.

The diagnosis is established by a tissue biopsy by an otolaryngologist. Blood testing can also reveal an elevated erythrocyte sedimentation rate and a positive anti-proteinase 3 antibody titer by enzyme-linked immunoabsorbent assay (ELISA) methodology. These are the blood tests that your physician should order if he or she believes that you suffer from Wegener's.

The treatment of this disorder is varied and includes chemotherapy with cytotoxic medication as well as steroids in addition to various immunosuppressives and different monoclonal antibodies. It is often difficult to keep the nose clean, so local care with frequent irrigation as well as an emollient is critical. Surgical treatment is generally geared on a symptomatic level, relieving pus, pain and pressure; and sinus surgery may be necessary to open up the areas to make them more accessible to relieve the crusting and infection.

For people with nasal and facial collapse, plastic surgery with grafting has become fairly successful. When I was consulting at the National Institutes of Health, we did research on different grafting techniques because of the poor success such patients had been experiencing. Dr. Robert Lebovics and I pioneered the use of certain types of grafts that have given patients new hope. These reconstruction efforts have met with much greater success than older procedures. Many patients experience problems with chronic eye tearing and require stents or even reconstruction of the tear ducts. Neodymiumyttrium-aluminum-garnet (YAG) laser helps burn through the bone via an intranasal approach, thus limiting the need for external surgery to repair the tear ducts. The repair of the tear ducts is known as dacryocystorhinostomy.

Churg-Strauss vasculitis is another disease that is similar to Wegener's. This disease is usually present with asthma and, necrotizing granulomata and vasculitis. Kidney disease is not present in Churg-Strauss, but Wegener's granulomatosis can cause renal failure. This can lead to decreased or absent urine production, and if left untreated, can cause mental status changes and even death. The signs, symptoms, and treatment of the sinonasal tract are similar with both Wegener's and Churg-Strauss. In Churg Strauss, people will also suffer from asthma, allergies, and have high eosinophilic counts on blood testing. In Wegener's, patients complain of shortness of breath, spitting up blood, pneumonia, and fever. A proper medical history is critical to differentiate between the two conditions.

Chronic Disorders and CAID

The following sections discuss chronic conditions that can make individuals more susceptible to infection, thus making them more prone to having problems with CAID. These patients require special treatment considerations. If you have been diagnosed with any of the following, there is a high probability that you may also suffer from CAID. Make sure to discuss your CAID symptoms with your primary-care physician as well as your specialists.

IMMUNOCOMPROMISED PATIENTS

If you have been diagnosed with an immunologic deficiency (like AIDS) or are currently on immunosuppressive therapy (including chemotherapy for arthritis or cancer), your CAID symptoms must be treated with special care. You might find that you are having more frequent sinus infections than before your illness. This may be due to the intrinsic illness or it may be due to the medications that you are taking, because many of them will lower your defense mechanisms.

As you know, you must be vigilant about your overall health: Even the smallest infection can lead to meningitis and/or periorbital infection (which can lead to visual changes or blindness). You will need to follow a preventative regimen and should consult an otolaryngologist as part of your treatment team. Once you have an ENT to advise you, he or she should provide you with a preventative regimen. The preventative regimen I give my immunocompromised patients is as follows:

- Take all medicines, including your sinus medicines religiously.
- Undergo daily nasal irrigation; twice daily if your sinus symptoms begin to flare.
- Seek immediate ENT medical attention as soon as you start to develop any sinus symptoms.

For years, many ENT surgeons were taught that sinus surgery wasn't advocated for people who also had AIDS, probably due to their perceived short life expectancy. But today's medicine has overcome this problem: AIDS patients are living longer, fuller lives and can benefit from sinus surgery. What's more, by following the preventative protocol, and treating sinus infections immediately as they occur, the need for surgery has become more limited as well.

CANCER PATIENTS

Radiation therapy that is delivered to the head and neck area can result in xerostomia, a chronic dry-mouth condition that is caused by damage to the salivary glands. You might also experience dryness to the mucous membrane in the nose and sinuses. The treatment protocol is very similar to the treatment of Sjögren's syndrome: frequent saline irrigation, emollients, nasal topical antibiotics, and nighttime humidifiers. Saline rinses are especially important because the normal mucociliary flow is often impeded after radiation therapy. This helps clean the nose and, in many individuals, decreases the amount of infection and crusting and thus makes the nose and sinuses feel more comfortable.

Radiation therapy or cancer itself may cause a change of taste or smell. Your sense of smell and taste can be temporarily or permanently altered, decreased, or may even disappear. Some people even report that they suffer from the presence of a foul sense of smell/taste. If you notice a severely decreased sense of smell, take extra steps to ensure safety around the home with smoke detectors and other appliances that can detect the presence of gas fumes or smoke in the home.

You may notice that even the foods you most enjoy now have a bitter taste or simply have less taste. The following suggestions may help make food taste better:

- Choose only the foods that continue to look and smell good to you.
- Serve foods at room temperature.
- Try using additional seasonings, including fresh herbs and spices.
- Try tart foods (such as oranges or lemons) that may have more taste, unless you are experiencing a sore mouth or throat.

DIABETES

It is widely believed that people with type 1 or type 2 diabetes are more prone to infection than their nondiabetic peers. Infection undoubtedly impairs blood sugar level control. For people with diabetes, controlling blood sugar levels not only is important for controlling the illness but also is necessary for treating subsequent infections and their complications.

The presence of diabetes impairs several aspects of white blood cell function, including cell movement. These people are prone to bacterial and fungal sinusitis with a greater frequency than the general public. They tend to suffer from chronic sinus infections and chronic pulmonary infections along with various other infections of other parts of their body. It is always harder to control recurrent sinus infections in diabetics. I explain to my patients with diabetes that it is of paramount importance that they be followed closely and that immediate action be taken when these infections flare. Furthermore, it is extremely important that they be compliant and take care of themselves in between infection flare-ups. It is also important that they work closely with their endocrinologist to keep their diabetes under control. For it is when the diabetes is out of control that they are most prone to the worst infections.

Lastly, people with diabetes are also prone to unusual infections with rare organisms. Bacterial and fungal infections can be very serious and complicated. Both acute and chronic bacterial and fungal sinusitis can lead to complications requiring immediate medical and sometimes surgical treatment. For example, bacterial infections in diabetics can spread to the eye, causing periorbital cellulitis (swelling of the eye socket contents), development of an abscess with protrusion of the eye, visual change and potentially blindness, or any combination of these symptoms. A bacterial infection can spread to the brain, leading to meningitis or a brain abscess. These complications can also happen to people who are not diabetic, although they are much more likely to occur with diabetics or immunocompromised patients.

RHINOCEREBRAL MUCORMYCOSIS

Rhinocerebral mucormycosis is a severe and potentially fatal fungal infection. This fungus typically affects people whose immune system is weakened by disease, such as uncontrolled diabetes, and/or AIDS. It is rarely found in someone with normal immune status. The symptoms of rhinocerebral mucormycosis include pain, fever, and an infection of the eye socket with a bulging of the affected eye. Pus is discharged from the nose. The roof of the mouth, the facial bones surrounding the eye socket or sinuses, or the nasal septum may be destroyed by the infection. Infection in the brain may cause seizures, partial paralysis, and coma. Because the symptoms of mucormycosis can resemble those of other severe bacterial infections, a doctor may not be able to diagnose it immediately. Usually the diagnosis is made when a doctor sees the organism in tissue samples. This is yet another reason why all immunocompromised patients should see an otolaryngologist who specializes in sinus problems as a part of their treatment team.

A person with mucormycosis is generally treated with intravenous antibiotics when there is a bacterial superinfection and with antifungal agents, like amphotericin B, given intravenously and/or injected directly into the spinal fluid. If tissue itself is infected, it needs to be removed by surgery.

LUPUS

Lupus is another autoimmune disease in which the body's defense mechanisms attack the body itself. It is thought to affect about 1 person in 1,000, with women nine times more likely to be affected than men. Although it can occur at any age, it usually appears in the late teens or early 20s.

Just about all parts of the body may be affected by lupus. Most often involved are the joints, the skin, the kidneys, the heart, and the lungs. Lupus is often treated with the same drugs used to treat malaria (hydroxychloroquine). Steroids may also be necessary. Sometimes drugs that suppress the body's immune system are used. I have seen many lupus patients suffering with CAID. The exact relationship between CAID and lupus is not known, but I suspect one exists.

CYSTIC FIBROSIS

Cystic fibrosis is a relatively rare inherited disease that affects the lungs and digestive system. The disease is chronic and progressive. In the past, it was believed that all cystic fibrosis patients succumbed to their disease by the age of 20. However, we are now finding that many of these people are living into their 50s and 60s. This may be because we now recognize more strains of the disease than we once did.

Because of the unique nature of this disease, it is critical that a team approach be used for long-term care and management. The team should include a pediatrician/internist, pulmonologist/cystic fibrosis specialist, anesthesiologist, and otolaryngologist. Cystic fibrosis causes the exocrine glands, which produce sweat and mucus, to produce abnormal secretions. This can include unusually thick, sticky mucus that clogs the sinuses and/or the lungs, leading to chronic respiratory problems. The disease can also affect the mucus that is secreted in various parts of the digestive tract, obstructing the ducts in the pancreas and preventing digestive enzymes from reaching the intestines to properly digest food. As a result, people with cystic fibrosis have trouble breathing and absorbing nutrients. They also have trouble eliminating waste. Nasal polyps are another common result of this disease. Some scientists believe that cystic fibrosis polyps are different from the nasal polyps formed in the general population. However, many of the same symptoms occur, including nasal airway obstruction, absent or decreased sense of smell, runny nose, and exacerbation of CAID. Medical therapy emphasizes relieving nasal obstruction with decongestants and topical nasal steroids, and using antibiotics when necessary to fight infection. Mucolytics, such as guaifenesin, and nasal saline sprays are also recommended. By loosening and eliminating nasal secretions, overall sinus drainage improves, and the probability of polyp buildup diminishes. The use of topical steroids has been shown to be beneficial for cystic fibrosis polyps as well. Nasal irrigation can be helpful in controlling infection and for clearing out the thick nasal secretions.

Surgical treatment is needed if there is a poor response to medical therapy. Between 10 and 20 percent of all cystic fibrosis patients will require surgical intervention for their sinus symptoms. Endoscopic surgical techniques allow for safe, minimally invasive surgery. Unfortunately, those with cystic fibrosis frequently suffer a recurrence of both nasal polyps and sinus disease. Interval antibiotic medical therapy slows the progression of disease, but frequent débridement and reoperation are usually necessary.

PATIENTS ON BLOOD THINNERS

Some people with congenital heart defects, including those that have had heart valve replacements, a stroke, a blood clot in the legs, or have had complicated surgeries may need to take daily anticoagulants, popularly known as blood thinners. These medicines slow blood clotting and are used to prevent major complications, such as vessel or valve obstruction or strokes. Blood thinners include aspirin and other anticoagulant medications such as Plavix and warfarin (Coumadin). Each of these medicines works on a different part of the blood-clotting cycle. There are also many over-the-counter (OTC) holistic products and vitamins that are used to retard clotting mechanisms. All of these agents can increase your risk of serious bleeding problems should you undergo surgery. It is important that you inform your surgeon that you are taking blood thinners before scheduling your procedure and to let your prescribing doctor know that you are considering surgery. Bleeding after surgery may be a serious complication of taking these medications. You will also need to monitor yourself very carefully after surgery. Tell your surgeon if you begin to bruise, have bleeding gums, or have nosebleeds. Serious bleeding after surgery could lead to days of nasal packing; a second trip to the operating room; the need for blood transfusions; and, in rare instances, even death. For patients currently taking warfarin and planning on having sinus surgery, I work with the treating physician, who will recommend one of the following:

- Discontinuation of warfarin 3–5 days before surgery
- Lowering the warfarin dose during the procedure
- Discontinuation of warfarin and treatment with intravenous heparin before and after surgery until the warfarin can be resumed

Special Needs for Every Generation

Each stage in life can also affect the course of treatment for CAID. Whether you are currently pregnant, in your later years, or caring for a child, read the following sections to make sure you are following the appropriate course of action.

PREGNANCY

As any pregnant woman can tell you, along with the complicated change in her hormones comes body swelling. The changes in a woman's body during pregnancy are designed to ensure the fetus adequate nutrition through the placenta and to protect the mother from trauma and blood loss at the time of delivery. Not only does a woman's body swell on the outside, but her nose and sinus membranes swell inside as well.

Endocrine and hormonal changes can also cause CAID symptoms. Most pregnant women experience hormonal changes, especially in the second and third trimesters, that may lead to nasal congestion. This is often very uncomfortable and occasionally leads to a sinus infection. The good news is that the swelling typically goes away within 1 week of giving birth. Aside from the usual symptoms of sinus disease, rhinitis (congestion) of pregnancy can cause sleep difficulty, including apnea in which oxygen saturation can drop and ultimately lower oxygen available to the fetus.

The management of CAID symptoms during pregnancy is controversial. Avoidance measures should be used first, especially if you already know that you have specific allergies or are sensitive to particular irritants. There are currently no CAID medicines that are considered absolutely safe during pregnancy, as most will cross the placenta. However, for severe cases, the following guidelines can be used under the supervision of a doctor's care:

- Decongestants can be used, although an overdose may interfere with the blood flow to the fetus.
- Nasal steroid sprays appear to be safe to use during pregnancy.
- Various medicines, including loratadine, cetirizine, budesonide, montelukast, nedocromil, lodoxamide, ipratropium, and cromolyn are in the U.S. Food and Drug Administration's Pregnancy Category B, which is defined as drugs that have not been shown to pose a risk to the fetus in studies in animals but that have not been adequately tested in pregnant women.
- It is not advised that pregnant women take any OTC remedies without physician guidance.

- Maintenance immunotherapy (allergy shots) may be safely continued during pregnancy if needed. Although immunotherapy is not known to harm the fetus, it is not a good idea to start such therapy during pregnancy. Immunotherapy doses are not increased and are often reduced until the postpartum period.
- Irrigation with nasal saline sprays, a neti pot, or a nasal irrigator is safe and effective to use during pregnancy.

Nursing mothers also need to pay particular attention to their sinuses. Treatment options are just as limited for nursing mothers as they are for pregnant women because some medicines will cross over from the mother's system and appear in the breast milk, which can have an adverse effect on the baby. Discuss any medicines that you take with your team of physicians, including your obstetrician-gynecologist (OB-GYN), pediatrician, and otolaryngologist. Together they should decide what you can take to treat your sinus disease.

I have had many patients who elected to have sinus surgery after their first pregnancy, because they did not want to suffer from recurring sinus infections in subsequent pregnancies. These are usually women who were treated for sinus problems before their first pregnancy and for whom surgery was recommended because medical therapy did not work. After surgery, and during their second pregnancy, most comment that they are glad that they went through with the surgery, because they did not experience the sinus discomfort that they experienced prior to surgery.

INFERTILITY

I believe that failure to conceive and carry a pregnancy to full term can be caused by changes in body temperature (low-grade fevers stemming from chronic sinus infections), drops in oxygen saturation, and the transient bacteremia that can occur with CAID. I've had a few female patients who have told me that they couldn't get pregnant until their sinus problems were resolved. Some underwent in vitro fertilization, which failed before resolving the sinus problem. After their sinus disease was cleared, these women successfully got pregnant—some without third-party assistance—and delivered healthy babies. I believe after speaking with various infertility specialists and endocrinologists that this is probably more common than is medically recognized.

If you are trying to conceive and are having difficulty with your sinuses, clear up any CAID issues before investing in expensive infertility treatments. Make sure your fertility specialist and your ENT communicate before, during, and after fertility treatment, so that you can receive the most comprehensive care.

OLDER PEOPLE

Many older men complain that their nose is constantly running. Others complain that their nose runs when they eat certain foods.

This symptom can be treated by your primary physician; however, these problems can be caused by a testosterone imbalance or by other endocrine disorders like hypothyroidism and gigantism. If you are suffering from this condition, it may be wise to consult with an otolaryngologist and an endocrinologist. There are various medicines that can also cause rhinitis with nasal discharge, and you should provide the entire list of medicines that you are taking because one of them may be the culprit of your nasal discharge.

Another sign of aging is that the mucous membranes may begin to dry. Some of my older patients complain that their nose often gets dry and crusty. Of the various disorders that may lead to a dry nose, one of the more common diseases is called Sjögren's syndrome. This is a chronic autoimmune disorder caused by an inflammatory attack of lymphocytes on the salivary glands. It is characterized by an exceedingly dry mouth and dry eyes. This loss of tear and saliva production may cause structural changes to the eyes and in the mouth. The nose may be affected as well. Often, those who suffer from this disease experience deterioration of the teeth due to cavities, increased oral infections, difficulty in swallowing, and a painful mouth. The blood of Sjögren's patients contains antibodies directed against normal cells. Therefore, this disease is termed an autoimmune disorder, to denote the reaction of the immune system against the patient's own tissues. The cause for this process remains unknown, but may be a virus.

Sjögren's usually occurs in middle-aged women. If you have been diagnosed with this disease, you may also have inflammation of the joints (arthritis), muscles, nerves (neuropathy), thyroid, kidneys, or other areas of the body. You may experience severe fatigue, and wake often during the night. Many Sjögren's sufferers complain of nasal dryness and have symptoms of sinusitis with postnasal drip. In my experience, people with Sjögren's do not get a higher frequency of sinusitis infections than other individuals. However, the infections tend to last longer and have a higher chance of developing into bronchitis or pneumonia. Diagnosis is based on clinical examination of the eyes and mouth. Specific blood tests and a biopsy taken from the inside of the lower lip help confirm the diagnosis.

Sjögren's syndrome is not fatal. However, you need to actively prevent possible complications due to dry mouth and dry eyes, as well as treatment of other organ systems involved as a consequence of the disease. My initial approach is to provide increased moisture to the eyes, nose, and mouth by use of nasal saline sprays during the day, and sleeping in a room with a humidifier at night. By rinsing the nose with a saline solution after loosening the secretions with a humidifier or in the shower, you can break the cycle of repeated sinus and upper-respiratory tract infections. There are many different types of cool-mist humidifiers that vary in size and cost. I recommend the smaller, portable units (choose one that is silent and easy to clean/refill) rather than large humidifiers that are added to a home's furnace/air-conditioning systems. The large room units may become contaminated with yeast or fungus that can subsequently irritate the sinuses. This problem is less likely to happen with the smaller units that can be cleaned and changed daily. In areas where the water is hard (contains large amounts of calcium and other salts), using distilled water may be less irritating and easier on the humidifier than water from the tap.

It is also important to keep the nose and sinuses clear, since mouth breathing can exacerbate the dry mouth problems associated with Sjögren's syndrome. In addition to the saline spray, it may be beneficial to irrigate the nose daily to remove dry, crusted, infected secretions. You can also try sucking candies and saliva substitutes, as well as eye drops that are recommended by an ophthalmologist. Medical options for treating severe cases of Sjögren's include steroids or other immune system suppressants. Patients with Sjögren's syndrome should create a medical team consisting of their primary-care physician, ophthalmologist, otolaryngologist, and rheumatologist in addition to any other practitioners who are treating them.

CHILDREN

CAID can affect children as well as adults. Very often, children are misdiagnosed by parents and well-meaning pediatricians as having yet another runny nose or just having a cold. Yet many of these children are congested all year long and are probably suffering from CAID.

A child's sinuses and nasal passageways are inherently smaller than an adult's and, therefore, are more easily obstructed. When children experience CAID symptoms, it usually stems from the fact that their sinuses have developed poorly: Their sinus passageways can be unusually small, or their small eustachian tubes are lying horizontally instead of at an angle. Often, their mouth is formed with a high arched palate. These children often breathe with a wide-open mouth, which is referred to as adenoidal facies.

All of these structural conditions can affect the child adversely. Due to constant infection and inflammation, his or her adenoidal bed is swollen and the tonsils are enlarged. Fluid will build up in the ears, leading to a secondary ear infection. Just as with adults, the child's sinus disease needs to be resolved before the ear infections will resolve. Furthermore, the underlying sinus disease will need to be resolved before the tonsil and the adenoidal infections will clear. Myringotomy, or ear tube placement, can temporarily solve the problem until the child's eustachian tubes grow larger in diameter and the angle becomes wider, allowing the eustachian tubes to drain the ears better, even in the face of continued chronic sinus infection.

The alteration of dentofacial structures may be caused by the child's inability to breathe through his nose. The constant mouth breathing influences the position of his tongue. As in all living things, form follows function. Bone growth is influenced by muscle function, thus the inability of the child to position his tongue appropriately against the dentofacial structures often has a detrimental affect on craniofacial development.

Recent peer-reviewed literature suggests that a time-tested device called the rapid palatal expander can enhance dentofacial development of these children. This device applies gentle pressure to the sutures of the palate in the mouth and the face and encourages new bone development, often aligning the nasal septum and expanding the palate and thus the floor of the nose. This allows children an improved ability to breathe. Recently, this device has been specifically recommended for children who are having difficulty breathing and sleeping at night. The device is fitted to the child's mouth through fixed orthodontic bands and can be inserted by the child or parent/guardian. Many of the children who received early treatment find that these expanders obviate the need for orthodontics later on because their dental growth is given positive direction by the expander.

Aside from structural issues, the most common symptoms that occur in children with CAID include swollen neck glands, cough, recurrent sore throats, enlarged tonsils, and recurrent strept infections, leading to many missed days of school. When children can't breathe and have chronic infections, they can experience bouts of recurrent bronchitis, pneumonia, tonsillitis, ear infections, and/or exacerbated asthma.

CAID vs. Tonsils and Adenoids

Tonsil and adenoid issues can also occur with chronic sinus infections with acute exacerbations. For kids with a constant yellow-green mucus and stuffy and runny nose, the infection can drain to the lymph nodes, which includes the neck nodes, tonsils, and adenoids. These children typically can't ever breathe through their nose.

A sinus infection with adenoidal enlargement in a child creates a vicious cycle. It is often difficult to tell which infection came first, and both eventually lead to a worsening of the other. For instance, a chronic sinus infection in a child can lead to swollen, infected adenoids, which leads to further nasal obstruction and then worsening of the sinus infection as the infected pus backs up. This constant nasal obstruction can lead to a sore throat, dry mouth, and worsening of a sinus infection.

Some pediatricians believe that this infection begins in the tonsils and adenoids and then backs up into the sinuses, but this makes no sense to me. Instead, I believe that the tonsils and adenoids become infected and swollen from the sinus infection. I call this secondary tonsillitis/adenoiditis. Most pediatricians and ENTs will decide to operate on the tonsils and adenoids without treating the sinus problem correctly. Unfortunately, many of these children are never treated by their pediatrician or their ENT with an antibiotic course longer than 2 weeks and neither the sinus nor the tonsil/adenoid infection clears. In my experience, many of these children would have improved without surgery had they been given a longer course of medicines.

For these children, I try the longer course of medications first. If their infections do not resolve within 3–8 weeks of antibiotics, then I recommend a CT scan of the sinuses. For children with a negative CT scan, I typically recommend another course of medical therapy. If this medical course fails, then I may consider surgery of the tonsils/adenoids.

There is a second type of tonsil and adenoid infection which I call primary tonsillitis/adenoiditis, in which the infection starts in the tonsils or in the throat, but these children typically have no problem breathing through their nose and won't have the yellow and green discharge that is common with a sinus infection. Typically, 2–4 weeks of antibiotics will resolve the infection. If this does not resolve with medication, your child may meet the criteria for tonsillectomy/adenoidectomy, depending on how many infections they have had in the past.

When coughing and wheezing are present in children, you may hear your doctor use the term *asthmatic bronchitis*. The coughing can be a barking, persistent cough with a wheeze, and the child may complain about tightness in his or her chest. These symptoms need to be addressed using the same methods that are used for treating adults. Typically, chronic sinusitis with asthmatic bronchitis requires a 3- to 8- (up to 12-) week course of antibiotics and other medicines. Usually when the sinus and nasal issues are resolved, the pulmonary conditions will clear. However, many pediatricians are reluctant to prescribe such a long course of medical therapy. Many parents are also afraid to give too many antibiotics to their children. However, undertreatment will only lead to recurring symptoms and infections.

Lastly, nasal obstruction and tonsillo–adenoidal (TA) enlargement can cause your child to snore or worse, suffer from sleep apnea. In recent studies, sleep apnea in children secondary to TA enlargement has been shown to affect daytime behavior, including inattention, hyperactivity, and/or sleepiness. Tonsillectomy and adenoidectomy in these children has been very effective in resolving sleep apnea. Furthermore, in these cases it has been shown that these children are significantly more likely to improve in their behavior and with their sleep problems.

CHAPTER 10

EAST MEETS WEST: COMPLEMENTARY HEALTH REMEDIES

Most classically trained physicians, including primary-care, allergists, pulmonologists, and otolaryngologists (including me) are starting to understand that chronic airway-digestive inflammatory disease (CAID) is caused by chronic inflammation and that the various diseases that make up CAID are connected. Yet practitioners outside of traditional Western medicine have always believed that the systems of the body are interconnected and that chronic inflammation plays a significant role in these disease processes. The practices associated with this philosophy have been somewhat haphazardly lumped together by the Western medical community as either "complementary," "alternative," "integrative," or Eastern medicine, which I use as a generic term for these practices. However, there are important distinctions among these individual philosophies: each group has its own ideas on the way the body works and how to best approach and address CAID symptoms.

In the war between traditional Western doctors and Eastern alternative practitioners, it appears that proponents are on one side or the other: Each group insists that you follow one type of practice while discarding the rest. Eastern practitioners were reluctant to accept Western ideas. Many Western practitioners disregarded these Eastern philosophies and their treatment modalities. Yet Western medicine can no longer deny their growing popularity. A recent study found that Americans made over 627 million visits to practitioners of alternative medicine in one year. A study by the Harvard Medical School found that one out of every two people between the ages of 35 and 49 regularly used at least one form of alternative treatment.

Today things are beginning to change. There are many classically trained physicians who have now incorporated complementary and alternative medicine (CAM) into their medical practices, providing the best of both worlds, and Eastern practitioners are now also working in concert with their Western allies. I am a proponent of the integration of these philosophies and treatments. Many medical schools now offer training in alternative medical approaches such as acupuncture, and many hospitals are starting to develop integrative medical centers. The prestigious National Institutes of Health has set up the Office of Alternative Medicine, and 34 medical schools in the United States have added elective courses in alternative medicine.

In my practice, I speak with practitioners from various Eastern philosophies on a daily basis, working together to provide my patients with the best care possible. I found that by tailoring a complementary program specific to each of my patient's needs, I can extract the best of all that is offered and provide the most comprehensive treatment, allowing the greatest chance of relief from symptoms. My patients often report great results with many alternative therapies, including osteopathic treatments, chiropractic care, acupuncture and acupressure, yoga, and natural remedies. In my mind, each of these treatment options has their place in CAID management and total sinus health. This chapter explains many of my Eastern colleagues' philosophies as they have been explained to me. I applaud these practitioners for bridging the gap between Eastern and Western medicine.

Remember, no one treatment will fit all people. Depending on your symptoms and diagnosis, some Eastern treatment options will be more successful than others. It is, therefore, still important to discuss these options with your traditional doctor, so that together you can determine which course is appropriate for you.

Acupuncture

Acupuncture originated in China more than 5,000 years ago and gradually spread across the entire Asian continent and to the West. It is believed to be the longest continuously practiced form of medicine in the world. In the United States, acupuncture's use has been on the rise since James Reston's landmark article describing his experience with postsurgical pain and acupuncture, which was published in the *New York Times* in 1971.

According to this medical philosophy, balanced health is determined by a flow of chi (pronounced *chee*), the vital life energy that animates all living beings. Chi flows to all parts of the body through 14 major energy pathways or meridians, 12 of which correspond to organs in the body. Chinese medicine attributes disease to an excess or deficiency of chi in different parts of the body, creating an imbalance. This imbalance can be caused by many factors, including heat, cold, dampness, emotions, diet, or exercise. Acupuncture tries to rebalance the flow of chi. In Western medical terms, chi may relate to the release of endorphins, the pain reliever naturally made by the brain, which has a calming effect.

A visit to an acupuncturist begins with a thorough medical history. Then the acupuncturist will perform a complete physical examination, taking note of the color of the skin, body language, and the tone of voice. The tongue is examined for color, the presence of a coating, or other irregularities that are believed to reflect overall health. Acupuncturists also focus on the body's pulse, which is felt at six locations since qualities of the pulse also reveal the balance and flow of chi.

Treatment begins by inserting sterile, hair-thin needles at selected points along the energy meridians. These needles alter the flow of chi by stimulating the specific points or by removing blockages. Acupuncturists often use additional modalities to stimulate acupuncture points, including heat, twirling of the needles, and electrical stimulation.

There are several types of acupuncture, each of which has proven to be effective.

1. Traditional Chinese medicine: favored in China and used in conjunction with herbal medicine
2. Medical acupuncture: performed by a traditional Western physician, which may incorporate other aspects of Western medicine
3. Japanese meridian acupuncture: uses thinner needles, which are placed more superficially
4. Five elements acupuncture: takes into account psychological components that might influence illness
5. Auricular (ear) acupuncture: based on the belief that the entire body can be treated by stimulating specific points on the outer ear.

HOW ACUPUNCTURE FEELS

Each individual will experience acupuncture differently. For most, acupuncture is relatively painless. You may be aware of a small discomfort once the needles are inserted, and you may experience a sensation of heaviness or mild aching after the treatment. This feeling is often desirable because it indicates that chi has been activated. Typically, results will be evident within six to eight treatments over a 2-month period, although chronic conditions may require longer therapy.

There are many certified physicians who have received additional medical training for acupuncture. You may want to contact the American Association of Medical Acupuncturists or a local acupuncture school or society for more information. There are other acupuncture practitioners who are outstanding, but because they have trained in China or other Asian countries, you may not be able to find them through traditional sources. Instead, you may be able to find them through acupuncture organizations or word of mouth.

ACUPUNCTURE AND CAID

Although acupuncture is most frequently sought as a treatment for physical pain such as back or neck ache, its traditional use is to treat a wide variety of conditions, ranging from gastroesophageal reflux disease (GERD) to allergies, asthma, and sinusitis. This is one of the many reasons I think it is an effective option for CAID sufferers. Among the conditions recommended for acupuncture treatment by the World Health Organization (WHO) are sinusitis, rhinitis, allergies, and asthma.

In traditional Chinese medicine, sinus symptoms are thought to be an invasion of external heat into the lungs, spleen, and stomach. Chronic cases are attributed to heat stagnating in the lungs or a deficiency of chi in the spleen. The spleen is considered to be the lung's mother: If there is a deficiency of chi in the spleen, the spleen cannot nourish the lungs.

The treatment of these symptoms would attempt to strengthen the spleen and remove excess heat. A traditional Chinese medical practitioner would prescribe nutritional therapy and add foods to your diet to clear heat and reinforce the spleen and lungs. Such foods include:

- Ginger
- Eggplant
- Pears
- Bananas
- Dates
- Yams

ACUPUNCTURE AND ASTHMA

Acupuncture has been shown to be effective in treating both acute and chronic asthma. In Chinese medicine, asthma is thought to be caused by external wind and cold influences or by excess heat, which is characterized by excessive sputum. The approach to dealing with asthma is relatively straightforward, with treatment directed toward the lung meridian as well as other points generally located on the chest and upper back. The kidney meridian is also related to asthma because it regulates the downward flow of chi and is used with greater frequency in childhood asthma, for which there is thought to be a greater deficiency of chi.

Acupressure

The difference between acupuncture and acupressure is that acupressure points are stimulated by hand rather than through the use of needles. There are a few useful techniques that can be done at home to alleviate symptoms of acute sinusitis.

You can apply pressure to some of the acupressure points the next time you have a sinus headache or infection. When using these points, apply a moderate amount of pressure and keep the pressure steady for 3–5 minutes until you feel the tension in the muscle relax or your pulse becomes smooth and steady. The most common points (Diagram 25) are as follows:

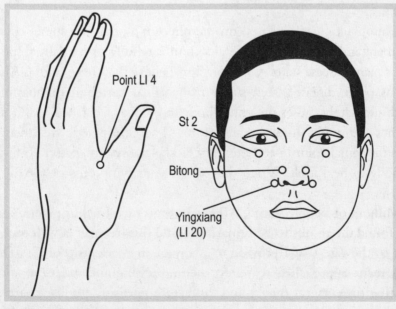

Diagram 25 Some common acupressure points.

- Large intestine 4 (li4): located in the webbing between your thumb and index finger
- Bitong: located at the base of the nasal bone, immediately above the junction of the lower lateral cartilage and the septum
- Large intestine 20 (li20): located lateral to the nasal alar at its widest point
- Stomach 2 (st2): small depression along the bone of the orbital rim, which is below the eye and directly below the pupil

Chiropractic Care

Chiropractic care is an alternative healing method for alleviating the nervous system from any interference, also known as subluxations of the spinal column. Both chiropractors and traditional medical practitioners agree that the nervous system acts as the body's communication center, sending messages from the brain to the rest of the body through nerve roots. These messages control our breathing, digestion, heartbeat, excretion, immune system function, glands, muscles, and countless other activities.

Chiropractic care is based on the philosophy that the spinal column alignment and the musculoskeletal system is wholly or partially responsible for many disease states. Chiropractors believe that those with CAID, as well as other disease states, suffer from spinal vertebral misalignment, which ultimately causes the entire body to be out of balance, manifesting as other seemingly unrelated symptoms. The chiropractic treatment realigns the spinal column and the musculoskeletal system, better equipping the body to heal itself. When this occurs your symptoms of CAID will clear.

Millions of people with CAID symptoms turn to chiropractic care. I have found the results to be remarkable, and this has been a welcome adjunct to the care that I provide to many of my patients. For CAID, the chiropractic approach is to relieve nerve pressure and inflammation by adjusting the cervical (neck) and thoracic (upper and midback) areas of the spine. During this adjustment, the bones of the spine are put gently back into proper alignment by the chiropractor. This will take any unhealthy pressure off of the spinal nerve roots thereby allowing the highway of communication to continue unimpeded. When the spine is returned to its proper alignment, many people experience symptomatic relief.

The adjustment is done in various ways, depending on the training of each particular chiropractor. Techniques include hands-on adjusting, use of an activator (an instrument that is placed on the bone and when pressed pushes the bone in place) or drop table, and the sacral-occipital technique. Many chiropractors use trigger-point therapy and/or yoga and stretching along with the adjustment to enhance the body's response and quicken the healing process.

Homeopathy

Homeopathy is a system of medicine that is widely practiced in Europe and is now finding its way around the world. I do not personally practice homeopathy, which requires specific training to accurately prescribe remedies. However, I often work with practitioners. Anecdotally, I have heard good reports. A study on the efficacy of homeopathic treatments has shown them to be more effective than taking a placebo. The success of homeopathy is based on a number of factors:

- Homeopathic remedies are completely safe and have no side effects or adverse interactions with other medications that you are taking.
- Homeopathy is based on completely natural ingredients.
- When the correct remedy is used, results are rapid and complete.
- Homeopathy does not suppress your immune system, it works in harmony with it.
- Homeopathic remedies attack the specific cause of your condition not the array of symptoms.

Like other forms of holistic treatment, homeopathy attempts to stimulate the body to repair itself. In general, homeopathic medicine is based on three principles.

1. Like cures like: Herbs that have a specific effect, when appropriately diluted, will have an opposing effect, as when an inoculation of viral particles stimulates the body to protect itself against further infection. For example, if arnica causes swelling then arnica, appropriately diluted, can also diminish swelling.
2. Minimal dose: Remedies are taken in an extremely diluted form, normally 1 part herb or other preparation in 6 or 10 million parts water.
3. A single remedy: Even if a number of symptoms are being experienced only one remedy will be prescribed, aimed at alleviating the entire complex of symptoms.

YOUR VISIT TO A HOMEOPATH

When you see a homeopath, he or she will take into account your constitutional type before prescribing a remedy. This means assessing a person's physical, emotional, and intellectual makeup as part of the diagnosis. Then a remedy will be prescribed and a course of action outlined.

I have found only two barriers to the use of homeopathic remedies. The first is that only the exact remedy can be prescribed for one's unique set of symptoms. For example, a remedy needs to be matched to a particular type of headache based on when it occurs, the type of pain, where it is located, and what other symptoms are associated with it. Therefore, it is important for you to find a holistic doctor who has the knowledge to correctly diagnosis your problem so that he or she can match up the appropriate holistic remedy (which can be one or a combination of various products). A proper holistic prescription works well but can take longer to determine than prescribing conventional medicines.

The second barrier is the sheer number of remedies available. Because of their unique nature, there are literally thousands of combinations of homeopathic remedies. Yet for practical purposes only the most common remedies can be carried by supermarkets or drugstores. To re-solve your particular problem, it might be difficult to find the exact holistic products that you need.

HOMEOPATHIC REMEDIES

Homeopathic medicines are products made by homeopathic pharmacies in accordance with the processes recognized by the U.S. Food and Drug Administration. The substances may be made from plants, minerals, animals, or even from chemical drugs. Each of these substances is diluted carefully until little or none of the original remains. Some of the most common remedies for CAID symptoms are as follows:

- **Hepar sulphuricum.** Used for later stages of sinus inflammation, when pain is behind the eyes and nasal discharge is thick.
- **Kali bichromicum.** Prescribed when there is pain between the eyes, on the forehead, or above one eye, accompanied by stringy nasal discharge. The scalp and facial bones are tender to the touch and pain is worse with cold and/or motion, and improves with warm compresses.
- **Mercurius.** Used for sinusitis with thick green nasal discharge or a gripping pain around the head extending to the teeth. Often, this pain worsens with open air, eating, drinking, and extremes of hot and cold.
- **Pulsatilla.** Prescribed for thick yellow discharge and is also associated with nausea and indigestion. Symptoms may improve with exposure to cool air or cool compresses and worsen when lying down, especially in a warm room.
- **Spigelia.** Given for sharp pain on the left side of the face after exposure to cold weather. Symptoms are aggravated by warmth, light noise, and movement and are relieved with cold compresses.
- **Silica 6c.** Used when pain begins in the back of the head and settles over the eyes.
- **Comb q.** Used for nasal discharge and general swelling of the sinuses.

- **Nat Mur 6c.** Used for a headache that begins at the root of the nose and extends to the forehead and is associated with nausea.

If you are interested in pursuing a homeopathic course of treatment, use the resources at the National Center for Homeopathy at www .homeopathic.org to find a qualified homeopathist in your city.

Osteopathic Medicine

Osteopathic medicine is also based on a philosophy that treats and heals the entire patient, as opposed to a crisis-oriented approach. Osteopathic philosophy stresses the importance of the body's own natural healing powers as well as the importance of the musculoskeletal system in general health. It is a truly holistic medical approach. Its founder, Andrew Taylor Still, was a Civil War surgeon who was discouraged by the overuse of medication during his day. He sought to develop a system of medicine that would restore the body's own natural defenses.

Today, osteopathic physicians are trained and certified throughout the United States and practice many of the same medical specialties as allopathic physicians (M.D.s). Their method seeks to use holistic approaches first and then medical or surgical treatment when needed. Osteopaths (D.O.s) are doctors licensed to practice medicine and surgery, in much the same way as their medical doctor (M.D.) counterparts. In addition to their traditional medical training, they also learn the art and science of manipulation. Manipulation is a method of treatment whereby the physician uses a hands-on approach to ensure that the body is moving freely and its innate healing systems can work unhindered.

OSTEOPATHY AND CAID

Studies in the United States and abroad have shown that osteopathic interventions can help CAID sufferers. In the case of sinusitis, osteopaths believe that the thick mucus produced in the sinuses is not adequately drained and the unequal pressure leads to pain. Because the nerves responsible for the sinuses begin in the thoracic (chest) area and pass through the neck, these areas would be evaluated and treated for any dysfunction through manual manipulation. Sinus headaches are another area known to respond well to this type of therapy.

Some osteopathic techniques can be done at home and are meant to relieve obstruction and pain. One technique involves pressure applied directly with the thumbs over the frontal sinuses and is gradually increased and released in a rhythmic manner. The thumbs are then placed in the center of the forehead and are gently moved laterally toward the temples, and downward toward the cheekbones (Diagram 26). This cycle is repeated 6–8 times. Next, one finger is placed at the brow directly above the nose (look for a small depression, called the supraorbital notch). Once located, pressure is applied with the thumbs, which are swept along the eye ridge laterally. This cycle is repeated 6–8 times.

The same technique is then applied to the maxillary sinuses. Pressure is applied over the sinuses with the thumbs beginning on each side

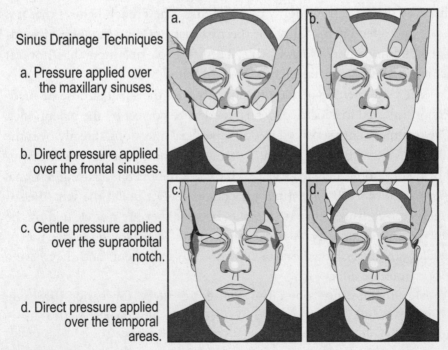

Sinus Drainage Techniques

a. Pressure applied over
   the maxillary sinuses.

b. Direct pressure applied
   over the frontal sinuses.

c. Gentle pressure applied
   over the supraorbital
   notch.

d. Direct pressure applied
   over the temporal
   areas.

Diagram 26

of the nose and pressing down while sweeping the thumbs along the maxilla (cheekbone). Then direct pressure is applied over the temples, with the area being compressed repeatedly in a gentle rhythmic motion.

If you are suffering from nasal congestion, place the thumbs on each side of your nose at the level of the bridge. Apply pressure alternately by each thumb moving down the length of the nose and sweeping laterally along the cheek. Although only one set of the sinuses may produce pain, the entire set of techniques should be performed to assist drainage as all the sinuses may be involved. I have also found osteopathic care to be helpful to many of my patients. I would recommend to those who are seeing an osteopath that they ask their practitioner to teach them the proper techniques for the pressure therapies I just described. To find an osteopathic physician, visit www.osteopathic.org.

MESOTHERAPY

Mesotherapy has been used in France for over 50 years and is recognized by the French Academy of Medicine. The French believe that it is a safe and effective modality for the treatment of a wide range of medical conditions, including CAID. This type of treatment has not yet achieved widespread acceptance in the United States.

The basic premise of mesotherapy is to use the smallest dose of medication, injected in a location determined to be correct by the practitioner. The treatment consists of a series of superficial injections, directly over the affected site, with conventional, botanical, or homeopathic medications. The medication is injected to a depth of 1–2 millimeters, causing minimal to no discomfort. By injecting intracutaneously, or under the skin, the solutions can remain in the area longer, because they are not cleared by the bloodstream as quickly as a deep injection. This allows for the use of smaller amounts of medication compared to oral agents and they have a more profound effect.

Mesotherapy can open the sinuses to allow for easier drainage. Usually a solution is prepared and injected locally over the affected sinuses. The solution is composed of three ingredients:

- **Procaine.** A local anesthetic that can dilate the blood vessels, allowing easier absorption of medications.
- **Pentoxifylline.** A medication that improves the properties of the blood flow, thereby enhancing tissue oxygenation. It also has been shown to inhibit neutrophil activation. (Neutrophils are the bloods inflammatory cells and are frequently present in chronic sinusitis.)
- **Calcitonin.** A parathyroid hormone that acts as a potent anti-inflammatory whenever bone is involved (as in the case of sinusitis).

I have patients who speak very highly about their success with mesotherapy. Often, these patients suffer from headaches (temporo mandibular joint, migraine, sinus) that have been hard to resolve with other forms of therapy. It is my understanding that there are very few mesotherapy practitioners in the United States.

Naturopathic Remedies

Naturopaths practice many of the techniques used by other practitioners and believe in healing by restoring strength to the individual rather than by curing specific diseases. They have a strong reverence for the healing power of nature. The goal for all practitioners of natural healing is to stimulate the body to heal itself. Rather than trying to attack specific diseases, natural healers focus on cleansing the body. Check with your local naturopathic society to find one near you.

Naturopaths often recommend the use of a neti pot. This ancient treatment, which I described in Chapter 4, provides gentle nasal irrigation. Naturopaths recommend adding a drop of tea tree oil into the saline solution, which they feel provides symptomatic relief while also inhibiting bacterial growth.

Hot baths and/or steam heat with a few drops of eucalyptus, peppermint, and/or tea tree oil are also a gentle way to initiate treatment. Naturopaths use lots of natural botanical extracts and vitamin/mineral supplements for various CAID symptoms and conditions, including:

- A multivitamin with B complex is suggested.
- Vitamin C and echinacea have been shown to boost the immune system and help fight off infection before it occurs. Conversely, low vitamin C intake is associated with a higher asthma risk in children. Vitamin C is an antioxidant.
- Zinc gluconate prevents viruses from implanting in the nasopharyngeal region.
- Gingerroot is used to make a powerful tea that provides symptomatic relief of nasal congestion and sore throat and is also rich in vitamin C. The steam from the ginger tea acts as an excellent cough suppressant.
- Ganmaoling is a popular Chinese herbal remedy that contains a minute amount of ephedra, which can raise your blood pressure and stress your circulatory system. This herb should be taken only with a doctor's supervision. It is more commonly used for acute sinusitis. It is never safe to use pure ephedra for CAID symptoms.
- Licorice root can help reduce bronchial inflammation and has expectorant effects.

Functional Medicine

Functional medicine blends biochemistry, anatomy, and naturopathy into an approach that is both conceptually and practically useful for the treatment of CAID. One of their key premises is that a leaky gut or increased intestinal permeability underlies chronic inflammation.

LEAKY GUT SYNDROME

Both functional and traditional physicians agree that the small and large intestines are lined by mucus cells linked together by bridges called desmosomes. This lining creates a barrier that is impermeable to all substances, allowing only electrolytes to move freely across the wall. This barrier prevents unwanted molecules from entering into our bloodstream.

Our body absorbs nutrients when larger proteins and carbohydrates are broken down into smaller units until they fit into receptors on the

cell's membrane, like a lock and key, and are actually engulfed by proto-
plasm from the cell. Nutrients can then be transported to our bloodstream and circulatory system. However, there are many factors that can
partially disrupt the desmosomes, allowing larger particles to pass
through this barrier or enter directly into the bloodstream before they
are adequately broken down. When this occurs, they are seen by the
body as antigenic, "foreign invaders," which sets off a low level inflammatory reaction meant to protect the body.

This low-grade inflammatory response is what functional medicine
believes is the key to understanding a host of conditions, ranging from
arthritis and eczema to chronic sinusitis and asthma. Factors that can disrupt the desmosomes fall into five common categories.

Food and Allergies

There are two types of allergies. The first is a sudden onset reaction, as
when someone with an allergy to ragweed is exposed to the allergen
and quickly develops a rash, shortness of breath, nasal congestion, and
sneezing. A second, more insidious form that usually goes unrecognized
is a delayed-onset reaction. In this form, the individual may notice only
some fatigue, bloating, "mental fog," or an exacerbation of chronic pain
and congestion. Exposure to the allergen may cause damage to the
desmosomes, allowing leaky gut syndrome to develop, thus deteriorat-
ing the body's defense against specific allergens. The liver, which is responsible for detoxifying the blood, is thus overwhelmed by the number
of foreign particles passing through what should have been an impermeable wall. The sufferer's sensitivity to that allergen increases because
it cannot be detoxified by an overwhelmed liver. Food sensitivities are
distinguishable from food allergies by their effect on the nonimmuno-
logical pathways in the body. Their effect is no less serious, however.
Conditions such as celiac disease, due to gluten sensitivity, or lactose intolerance can dramatically influence leaky gut disorders.

Dysbiosis

The gut normally maintains a balance of different types of bacteria. The
good bacteria are symbiotic: They help digest food and form substances

such as butyric acid, the "fuel" for the cells lining the gut wall. The bad bacteria are usually held in check by the large numbers of good bacteria, which are able to get to most of the ingested food before the bad bacteria, in effect controlling their population growth by limiting their food supply. The good bacteria continue to grow, while the population of bad bacteria remains small. When this balance is disrupted, it is called dysbiosis, which can be caused by a long course of antibiotics, allowing the bad bacteria to flourish. The toxins produced by the bad bacteria may cause damage to the gut walls as well. In addition, the cells that line the gut wall are deprived of the needed byproducts of the symbiotic bacterial metabolism, byproducts the cells need to thrive.

Infection

An active infection by a parasite, fungus, or bacterium can wreak havoc on the gut lining. *Candida* or yeast-related disorders can also wreak havoc in the body. There are numerous diets and theories about yeast infections in the gut, and how they weaken the immune system. These are intimately related to fungal conditions elsewhere in the body.

Anti-inflammatories

Frequent use of nonsteroid anti-inflammatory drugs, such as naproxen (Aleve), ibuprofen, and aspirin can also adversely affect the gut wall.

Alcohol

Large amounts of alcohol can damage the gut. This can be quantified as more than 1 glass of wine or beer a day for women, 2 for men.

COURSES OF ACTION

(Functional medicine advocates refer to this as the 4 Rs.)

1. *Remove*: Eliminate infections that are found. Stop taking anti-inflammatories and drinking excess alcohol. Begin an allergy elimination diet, which removes toxins in food that may trigger

an inflammatory response. (The elimination diet is given at the end of the chapter.)

2. *Replace*: Add fiber, digestive enzymes, and hydrochloric acid to the diet to restore balance and homeostasis to the gastrointestinal (GI) tract.

3. *Repair*: Take a number of anti-inflammatory herbs, nutrient vitamins, and antioxidants to repair the gut lining.

4. *Reinnoculate*: Reintroduce the symbiotic bacteria by taking probiotics, such as bifidus, acidophilus, or saccharomycosis boulardi, alone or in combination.

NUTRIENTS AND HERBS

The following list includes only a few of the substances that functional medicine practitioners use for CAID symptoms. They believe that if taken daily, these nutrients will reduce symptoms and restore a normal intestinal permeability.

- **Probiotics.** As mentioned in Chapter 4, these helpful bacteria are crucial for intestinal health. They are even more crucial for treating CAID, for which antibiotics are extensively used.

- **Glutamine.** L-glutamine is a fuel for the cells of the colon and small intestine and provides energy for the rapidly dividing cells of the immune system. Without glutamine, the gut cells cannot reproduce.

- **Zinc.** Zinc may be useful in fighting viral infections. Many functional medicine practitioners believe that a significant number of the population is deficient in zinc.

- **Bee pollen and propolis.** Bee pollen is produced by the anthers of flowering plants and is gathered by bees. Propolis is a collection of various plant secretions that act as a binding substance for beehives. Both are reported to be effective for people with allergies, as they provide the enzymes and complex proteins needed to restore damaged cells within the immune system. Both also reduce the inflammatory response from overproduction of histamines.

- **Berberine.** The active ingredient found in goldenseal, an herb native to North America, berberine has important antibacterial and antifungal effects.
- **Butyrate.** A short-chained fatty acid produced in the colon by a fermentation of fiber, butyrate is a major source of fuel for the colon's cells.
- **Curcumin.** A chemical found in tumeric (a spice used in curry), curcumin has been found to be a potent anti-inflammatory as well as having a beneficial effect on the liver, stimulating the flow of bile and the breakdown of fat.
- **Essential fatty acids (EFAs).** These fats cannot be produced by the body but must be supplemented in one's diet. There are two types of EFAs: omega-6 and omega-3. Omega-3s are found primarily in fish and are known to reduce leukotrienes, which are found in the cells responsible for inflammation. They also increase the activity of killer cells, which are critical to fighting infection and controlling the proliferation of cancer cells. Omega-3s help normalize the immune system, have been successfully used to treat many chronic inflammatory conditions, and are specifically useful in chronic sinusitis. To ensure the safety of fish oil supplements, always check to see that the label says "pharmaceutical grade" to be certain that the supplements have been cleared of residual mercury or cadmium. Omega-6s are primarily found in plant based oils. There are "healthy" omega-6 fatty acids found in primrose oil. There is increasing evidence that deficiencies of omega-3 fatty acids and increases in omega-6s found in margarine and fried food have contributed to inflammatory conditions, such as asthma. A balance between omega-3 and omega-6 is crucial for a healthy body.
- **Gingerroot.** Ginger contains an enzyme that increases the digestion of protein. It is used to relax the smooth muscle of the intestines. Ginger also inhibits leukotrienes, the cells that trigger inflammation.
- **N-Acetylcysteine (NAC).** NAC is useful for enhancing liver detoxification, pulmonary function, and intestinal health. This

amino acid is also produced naturally by the body. It is converted to glutathione, which is a crucial antioxidant and is the primary agent used by the liver for detoxification.

- **Niacinamide.** This form of vitamin B increases the levels of anti-inflammatory enzymes, which is useful in chronic sinusitis.
- **Quercitin.** A bioflavonoid found in the skin of red apples and in the skin of all onions, quercitin is a natural antihistime and an effective remedy for allergies. It has important anti-inflammatory effects and stabilizes mast cells, the cells that release histamines. It is also a potent antioxidant and can calm an overactive immune system.
- **Vitamin A and beta-carotene.** Most vitamin A comes from the precursor beta-carotene, which is converted to vitamin A in the GI tract and is vital to maintaining the integrity of mucous membranes that line the sinuses and respiratory tract. Beta-carotene is found in yellow, orange, and red fruits and vegetables, such as carrots, yams, cantaloupe, peaches, and papayas. Vitamin A can be taken directly as a supplement from cod liver oil, but due to the danger of toxicity and its link to osteoporosis at high doses, it should be supplemented only under medical supervision.

Pregnant women are advised against taking all of the above supplements.

DIET CAN BE A SOLUTION

The "remove" aspect of functional medicine (the first of the 4 Rs) includes dietary changes, particularly when there has been a history of antibiotic misuse. When necessary, I send patients to holistic practitioners who prescribe the following allergy elimination diet as a way to cleanse my patients' internal systems before more aggressive treatment, including prescription medications or surgery is initiated. This type of diet eliminates—for 2–3 weeks—most foods that have been commonly found to be allergenic. Afterward, foods can be reintroduced into the diet individually so patients can see whether any of them cause an exacerbation of symptoms. If symptoms worsen, the food group is then avoided.

Caffeine and alcohol are usually removed, as well as dairy, wheat, corn products, and the night shade vegetables (which include eggplants and tomatoes). These are the primary food groups that should be eliminated, but following a complete elimination diet is preferable.

I also tell my patients to avoid all white sugar and white flour. These products depress the immune system and support the life cycle of fungal organisms. Initially, many people have difficulty finding foods that satisfy them, but the results are so reinforcing that it soon becomes a way of life. A good-quality, broad-spectrum probiotic replacement is also essential.

COMPREHENSIVE ELIMINATION DIET

This is called an "elimination diet" because you will be removing certain foods and food categories from your diet. These modifications allow your body's compromised detoxification machinery to recover and begin to function efficiently. The dietary changes help the body eliminate or "clear" various toxins that may have accumulated due to environmental exposure, foods, beverages, drugs, alcohol, or cigarette smoking. This is not a calorie-restricted diet.

I find that those patients who can follow the diet report increased energy and mental alertness, decreased muscle or joint pain, and a general sense of well-being. However, some people do not tolerate the change in diet well. Don't be surprised if you experience changes in sleep patterns, lightheadedness, headaches, joint or muscle stiffness, and changes in gastrointestinal function during the first week. The good news is that these symptoms rarely last for more than a few days.

INSTRUCTIONS FOR THE COMPREHENSIVE ELIMINATION DIET

Eat only the foods listed under "Foods to Include" and avoid foods listed under "Foods to Exclude." If you have a question about a particular food, check to see if it is on the food list. Avoid any of the permissible foods if you know you are intolerant or allergic. Pay attention to the following guidelines as you choose your foods each day:

- You may use leftovers for the next day's meal or part of a meal (e.g., leftover broiled salmon and broccoli from dinner as part of a large salad for lunch the next day).
- It may be helpful to cook extra chicken, sweet potatoes, rice, and beans, etc. that can be reheated for snacking or another meal.
- Most foods on the menu plan freeze quite well.
- Please add extra vegetables and fruits as needed. The menu is a *basic* one and needs your personal touch. Use the suggested snacks as needed for hunger or cravings; leftovers are also handy to eat as snacks.
- If you are a vegetarian, eliminate the meats and fish and consume more beans and rice, quinoa, amaranth, teff, millet, and buckwheat.
- Breakfasts that need cooking are easiest to incorporate on your days off. Muffins can be made ahead of time, frozen, and used as needed.
- If you are consuming coffee or other caffeine containing beverages on a regular basis, it is always wise to slowly reduce your caffeine intake rather than abruptly stop it; this will prevent caffeine-withdrawal headaches. For instance, try drinking half-decaf/half-regular coffee for a few days, then slowly reduce the total amount of coffee.
- Select fresh foods whenever you can. If possible, choose organically grown fruits and vegetables to eliminate pesticide and chemical residue consumption. Always wash fruits and vegetables thoroughly.
- Read oil labels; use only those that are obtained by a "cold pressed" method.
- If you select animal sources of protein, look for free-range or organically raised chicken, turkey, or lamb. Trim visible fat and prepare by broiling, baking, stewing, grilling, or stir-frying. Cold-water fish (e.g., salmon, mackerel, and halibut) is another excellent source of protein and the omega-3 essential fatty acids, which are important nutrients in this diet. Fish is used extensively. If you do not tolerate fish, consult with [your physician/health-care practitioner].

Supplemental fish oils may be suggested. Avoid shellfish, as it may cause an allergic reaction.

- Remember to drink the recommended amount (at least two quarts) of plain, filtered water each day.
- Strenuous or prolonged exercise may be reduced during some or the entire program to allow the body to heal more effectively without the additional burden imposed by exercise. Adequate rest and stress reduction are also important to the success of this program.

Note that, any time you change your diet significantly, you may experience symptoms such as fatigue, headache, or muscle aches for a few days. Your body needs time as it is "withdrawing" from the foods you eat on a daily basis. Your body may crave some foods it is used to consuming. Those symptoms generally don't last long, and most people feel much better over the next couple of weeks.

Comprehensive Elimination Diet Guidelines
TABLE 2. ELIMINATION DIET

FOOD CATEGORY	FOOD TO INCLUDE	FOODS TO EXCLUDE
Fruits	Whole fruits, unsweetened frozen, water-packed canned fruits, diluted juices	Oranges, orange juice
Dairy substitutes	Rice, oat, and nut milks (almond milk and coconut milk)	Milk, cheese, eggs, cottage cheese,cream, yogurt, butter, ice cream, frozen yogurt, nondairy creamers
Nongluten grains and starch	Brown rice, millet, quinoa, amaranth, teff, tapioca, buckwheat, potato flour	Wheat, corn, barley, spelt, kamut, rye, triticale

FOOD CATEGORY	FOOD TO INCLUDE	FOODS TO EXCLUDE
Animal protein	Fresh and water-packed fish, wild game, lamb, duck, organic chicken and turkey	Pork, beef/veal, sausage, cold cuts, canned meats, frankfurters, shellfish
Vegetable protein	Split peas, lentils, legumes	Soybean products (soy sauce, soybean oil in processed foods; tempeh, tofu, soy milk, soy yogurt, textured vegetable protein)
Nuts and seeds	Walnuts; sesame, pumpkin, and sunflower seeds; hazelnuts; pecans; almonds; cashews; nut butters (almond and tahini)	Peanuts, peanut butter
Vegetables	All, raw, steamed, sautéed, juiced, or roasted	Corn, any creamed
Oils	Cold-pressed olive, flax, safflower, sesame, almond, sunflower, walnut, canola, pumpkin	Butter, margarine, shortening, processed oils, salad dressings, mayonnaise, spreads
Drinks	Filtered, distilled, seltzer, and mineral water; decaffeinated herbal tea	Alcohol, coffee and other caffeinated beverages, soda pop (soft drinks)
Sweeteners	Brown rice syrup, agave nectar, stevia, fruit sweetener, blackstrap molasses	Refined white and brown sugar, honey, maple syrup, high-fructose corn syrup, evaporated cane juice

FOOD CATEGORY	FOOD TO INCLUDE	FOODS TO EXCLUDE
Condiments	Vinegar, all spices and herbs	Chocolate, ketchup, relish, chutney, soy sauce, barbecue sauce, teriyaki sauce, other condiments

Things to Watch For

- Corn starch in baking powder and any processed foods
- Corn syrup in beverages and processed foods
- Vinegar in ketchup, mayonnaise, and mustard is usually from wheat or corn
- Breads advertised as gluten-free that contain spelt, kamut, or rye
- Many amaranth and millet flake cereals have corn
- Many canned tunas contain textured vegetable protein that is from soy; look for low-salt versions, which tend to be pure tuna, with no fillers
- Multigrain rice cakes are not just rice; purchase plain rice cakes

Elimination Diet Shopping List

FRUITS*
Apples, applesauce
Apricots (fresh)
Bananas
Blackberries
Blueberries
Cantaloupe
Cherries
Coconut
Figs (fresh)
Grapefruit
Huckleberries

Kiwi
Kumquat
Lemon
Lime
Loganberries
Mangos
Melons
Mulberries
Nectarines
Papayas
Peaches
Pears

Prunes
Raspberries
Strawberries
* All these fruits can be consumed raw or juiced.

VEGETABLES†
Artichoke
Asparagus
Avocado
Bamboo shoots
Beets and beet tops

Bell peppers
Bok choy
Broccoflower
Broccoli
Brussels sprouts
Cabbage
Carrots
Cauliflower
Celery
Chicory, red leaf
Chives
Cucumber
Dandelion greens
Eggplant
Endive
Kale
Kohlrabi
Leeks
Lettuce, red or green
   leaf and Chinese
Okra
Onions
Parsley
Potato
Sea vegetables, seaweed
   and kelp
Snow peas
Spinach
Squash
Sweet potato (yams)
Swiss chard
Tomato
Watercress
Zucchini
† *All these vegetables*
can be consumed raw,

juiced steamed, sautéed,
or baked.

BEANS (DRIED OR
CANNED)
All except soy
Lentils, brown, green,
   red
Split peas

NUTS AND SEEDS‡
Almonds
Cashews
Flax seeds
Hazelnuts (filberts)
Pecans
Pistachios
Poppy seeds
Pumpkin seeds
Sesame seeds
Sunflower seeds
Walnuts
‡ *All these seeds and*
nuts can be consumed as
butters and spreads
(e.g., tahini).

NONGLUTEN GRAINS
Amaranth
Buckwheat
Millet
Oat
Quinoa
Rice, brown, white, and
   wild
Teff

VINEGARS
Apple cider
Balsamic
Plum
Red wine
Rice
Tarragon

HERBS, SPICES, AND
EXTRACTS
Basil
Black pepper
Cinnamon
Cumin
Dandelion
Dill
Dry mustard
Garlic
Ginger
Nutmeg
Oregano
Parsley
Rosemary
Salt-free herbal blends
Sea salt
Tarragon
Thyme
Turmeric
Vanilla extract, pure

CEREALS AND PASTA
Buckwheat noodles
Cream of rice
Oats
Puffed millet
Puffed rice

Quinoa flakes
Rice crackers
Rice pasta

BREADS AND BAKING
Arrowroot
Baking soda
Flours, rice, teff, quinoa,
   millet, tapioca,
   amaranth, garbanzo
   bean, potato,
   tapioca
Gluten-free breads
Mochi
Rice bran
Rice flour pancake mix

FLESH FOODS
Free-range chicken,
   turkey, duck
Fresh ocean fish, Pacific
   salmon, halibut, had-
   dock, cod, sole, pol-
   lock, tuna, mahi-mahi

Lamb
Tuna, water-packed
   canned (watch for
   added protein from
   soy)
Wild game

DAIRY SUBSTITUTES
Almond milk
Coconut milk
Oat milk
Rice milk

**BEVERAGES,
NONDAIRY**
Fruit juices, pure,
   unsweetened
Herbal tea, noncaf-
   feinated
Mineral water
Spring water
Vegetable juices, pure,
   unsweetened

OILS
Almond
Canola
Flax seed
Olive
Pumpkin
Safflower
Sesame
Sunflower
Walnut

SWEETENERS
Agave nectar
Fruit sweeteners,
   apple juice
   concentrate
Molasses
Rice syrup
Stevia

CONDIMENTS
Mustard, made with
   apple cider vinegar
Nutritional yeast

ASTHMA AND FUNCTIONAL MEDICINE

Functional medical practitioners believe that a low level inflammatory state contributes to bronchial irritability and the likelihood of bronchospasm. An analysis of 2,000 children showed that 80 percent had decreased acid output, suggesting that these children may have been predisposed to food allergies. These allergies may increase gut permeability, thus both increasing the level of inflammation as well as increasing the number of bronchostrictive compounds that enter the circulatory system.

Functional medicine therefore believes that the elimination diet is equally important for those who may think they are suffering from either asthma or food allergies. In addition, functional medicine practitioners believe that it is important to eliminate food additives, the artificial dyes and preservatives that are frequently added to foods. Sulfites, for example, are a well known agent that causes bronchoconstriction. They can be found in wine, beer, and the salads and vegetables that are served in restaurants. There is also evidence that histamine and bronchial reactivity to histamines increases with salt intake.

There are also many supplements that may be used to control asthma. For example, there is evidence that children with asthma may have a defect in the metabolism of tryptophan, thus a tryptophan-restricted diet or pyridoxine supplementation to correct the defect may be beneficial. Reduced selenium levels have been demonstrated in asthma patients, and selenium levels are critical to maintaining glutathione levels. This is, in turn, important in reducing leukotriene levels, inflammatory proteins that are responsible for bronchial reactivity. Selenium supplementation thus seems warranted, as well as supplementation with magnesium (a smooth muscle relaxant), a good antioxidant, Quercitin, and high levels of fish oil.

The future of medicine needs to incorporate all available modalities. Although we still have a great deal to learn about the disease processes described in this chapter, interested individuals now have a wide variety of resources available to help them in their pursuit of health.

CHAPTER 11

MOLD: THE LATEST RESEARCH, CAUSES, AND CURES

When I was asked to talk about mold on a nationally syndicated television show along with celebrity advocate Bianca Jagger, I realized that one of the hottest topics in medicine today had reached consumer consciousness. Mold was becoming an everyday problem: infiltrating our homes, schools, and workplaces. It was literally making people sick, and the public needed to know why. Because of my expertise, I was invited to explain one of the most pervasive health problems we are all facing today.

There are millions of types of naturally occurring molds in the world, and most of them can be considered as beneficial. Molds are used in making antibiotics, including penicillin and other medicines. Mold is also found in many of the foods we eat: We use it to ferment alcohol, beer, and vinegar, and to make bread (yeast), and to make a malted. Many types of fungi (another word for molds) normally live in our bodies: in the nose, sinuses, lungs, and in the gut. Generally, people do not react to these organisms. However, when this internal mold gets out of control, or if our bodies create an inflammatory response to this mold, significant health problems can result.

Mold can cause devastating systemic problems. Usually, it is the subsequent inflammatory process, and not the actual mold, that makes us sick. However, excessive mold growth can lead to a variety of health issues, from athlete's foot to jock itch, to fingernail or toenail mold, to fungal sinusitis. Though extremely rare, mold infections can invade the brain.

Mold and CAID

I have always believed that sinus disease was caused by both bacteria and fungus. Now, the latest scientific research proves that mold is a major cause of chronic airway-digestive inflammatory disease (CAID). It not only leads to sinus disease, it can affect each of the limbs that are connected to this disease process. Mold can trigger lung problems, including asthma. The inflammatory process spawned by a reaction to mold is also responsible for reactions in the upper and lower digestive tracts, affecting gastroesophageal reflux disease (GERD) and other stomach ailments. Mold can cause allergic reactions as well, further contributing to CAID. The connection between mold and sinus problems is so profound that it is forcing researchers to rethink the entire disease process, beginning with creating a new definition for sinus disease and chronic rhinosinusitis.

The term *rhinosinusitis* means "inflammation of the nose and sinuses." Traditionally, doctors and researchers believed that this inflammation was caused solely by bacterial infection, which could then be treated by antibiotics. The relationship between poor health and mold was inconclusive and thought to be limited to fungal allergies that were present in less than 10 percent of cases. However, recent studies indicate that fungus is likely the cause of nearly all chronic rhinosinusitis.

In 1999, a team from the Mayo Clinic headed by Jens Ponikau, David Sherris, and Eugene Kern shed tremendous light on this subject. Using new techniques for culturing mucus samples, they proved that 96 percent of the patients they tested were found to be culture positive for fungi that were causing CAID symptoms. The most common offenders were *Candida albicans*, *Alternaria*, *Penicillium*, *Cladosporium*, and *Aspergillus*. On average, most patients had more than two types of fungus present in their mucus, and some patients had up to eight. What's more, even normal, healthy individuals—those patients who did not have symptoms of chronic rhinosinusitis also cultured positive for the same fungi as patients with chronic rhinosinusitis. In fact, they found that almost everyone seemed to culture positive for fungi! So why then would fungus affect some and not others?

Ponikau, Sherris, and Kern determined that the difference seemed to be in the immunological response that each individual had toward mold. They proved that there is an immune-mediated response, different from an allergy, which occurs in people who react to the mold present in their body. This immune response starts off with a white blood cell called a lymphocyte, which secretes a substance called cytokines. When a fungus is in the vicinity of a lymphocyte, in mold-sensitive patients, it will produce and secrete two types of cytokines, which enlist other white blood cells (called eosinophils) to prepare themselves to attack the fungus, which is seen as a foreign invader to the body. Once eosinophils are called on by the lymphocyte, the eosinophils accumulate tiny granules of toxic material called major basic protein. Another cytokine activates the eosinophils to secrete the major basic protein and fight off the mold.

This all seems like a great mechanism for the body to rid itself of fungi. However, once the major basic protein is secreted, it has toxic effects on the delicate mucous membrane of your sinuses and nose, causing swelling and erosion—an inflammatory response. Once this occurs, the cilia that normally push the mucus out of the nose and sinuses cease to function. The mucus pools and then bacteria can multiply and cause the infection to fester. Furthermore, the major basic protein causes erosion of the membranes, allowing bacteria to freely invade the mucous membrane, causing further inflammation and infection. The bone underlying the sinus lining can become infected, called osteitis. The membranes of the sinuses swell and can start to form polyps.

Based on this study, scientists now believe that chronic rhinosinusitis is not only a direct result of the bacteria entering the nasal and sinus membranes but an indirect result of the immune response to fungi. More to the point, they believe that this is an abnormal response: They found that healthy patients lacked this immune response and, therefore, do not have the same reaction to fungi.

With this new knowledge comes many more questions and different views on what these data actually mean. We still do not know why some patients have an abnormal response to fungi. Some researchers are now studying whether the fungus reaction is really abnormal or whether it is a defense against a worse disease like cancer. For example, recent research has shown that children with asthma have a lower incidence of developing brain tumors. Maybe on some level, the mold in our systems protects us from other health issues. The answers still await us.

This research has given us the tools to determine if your sinus and nasal problem is due to an immune response to fungi. A new test has been developed that identifies the presence of major basic proteins in the mucus and/or a high concentration of eosinophils. This technology is now becoming available, but requires a visit to an ear, nose, and throat (ENT) physician specializing in nasal and sinus disorders.

Because I believe that CAID is probably caused by both the response to fungus and the bacterial infection that follows, I choose to treat both the bacteria and the fungus. If we can return the balance of the bacterial and fungal flora to normal, control the abnormal response to the fungi that has been identified through this research, and repair the membrane breach that occurs as a result to the toxins, we will be able to improve the control of sinus disease and make you feel better.

Increasing Fungus Sensitivity

It is not really known why people develop sensitivity to fungi. Some researchers believe that it is a result of extensive use of antibiotics, which can cause an overgrowth of mold. Others believe that antibiotic use has nothing to do with it. In my practice, I've seen firsthand that some people can be on antibiotics for the long term and have no fungal problems, while others take one or two pills from a single course of antibiotics and immediately develop a fungal or yeast infection. This sensitivity is certainly genetically programmed into each and every one of us. With this in mind, it may be useful to take probiotics, such as acidophilus, when taking antibiotics long term to help maintain the balance your body requires.

The Next Culprit: Fungal Infections

Scientists and doctors used to think that there were three variations of fungal infection. The first was labeled as topical, the second was locally invasive, and the third was systemically invasive. The newest research shows that they are really very similar. We now know that locally invasive fungus is simply fungus that has actually invaded the membranes and the bone. When the same fungus invades adjacent areas, including the brain, the orbit, or the blood vessels then it becomes systemically invasive.

Allergic to Mold

Fungal allergies may be a result of extensive exposure to mold and fungi in the environment. This can be due to both wet surfaces and more energy-efficient homes with less air exchange. All molds can affect the breathing system by causing two distinct internal reactions, either an immunologic inflammatory reaction or an allergic reaction. Many patients suffer both simultaneously. The allergic reaction occurs in the same manner as it occurs when allergic people are exposed to pollens and dusts. Almost half of all patients who have allergic fungal sinusitis also have a positive allergy skin test for fungi or mold. The immunologic reaction occurs similarly to the way that the body fights infection. The former can be as mild as itching and swelling and as severe as anaphylactic shock, although rare. The latter can be as mild as slight congestion to a severe asthma flare-up, or the response one would experience with a severe infection, all the way to a fight for life during invasive fungal sinusitis with a brain abscess.

MOLD

Ask yourself the following to see if you are allergic to mold:

- Do you sneeze or feel stuffy when you walk into a damp or musty house or basement or a damp barn or garage? Outdoor molds are a problem when raking or walking through or playing in the leaves in the autumn. Fallen leaves become moldy very quickly. If you enjoy camping or sleeping outdoors, mold allergies may be a problem, especially when it rains and is wet or in the fall.
- Do you feel sick when you return to or clean out a summerhome or old cabin after it has been closed for a season or two?
- Do you feel sick when around hay in the barn or on hayrides? Often there is a considerable amount of mold around hay and cut grass.
- Do plants or the garden make you feel stuffy? Often there is a lot of mold around our gardens because the soil is moist.
- Do damp seasons cause you to feel miserable? Although most molds grow outside, indoor molds grow near wet areas like garbage bins, food storage areas, in wallpaper, and in any area with increased humidity, such as damp basements, washrooms, bathrooms, kitchens, and rooms where there has been a leak and moisture persists. Carpeting and floor mats are excellent places for molds to grow when they are damp. Damp windowsills and bookcases are also attractive to mold.

Avoidance and reducing exposure to mold are the best ways to help prevent allergic reactions.

But as we've seen, fungal sinusitis is not merely an allergic phenomenon. It now appears that fungal sinusitis, once thought to be a rare disease in patients with severe immunological deficiencies, is much more common in patients who appear to have normal immunity. These people have a predisposition causing their bodies to have an inflammatory reaction to the mold. For example, many people experience sinus pain and infections in the fall: It is now thought that these seasonally signaled infections are due to mold caused by exposure to decaying leaves. Whether the reaction is immunologic or allergic, and it can be both, people need to be aware of these triggers and how to treat them most effectively.

It may be possible to treat mold allergies by using allergy desensitization management (allergy shots). Although it is virtually impossible to test for all types of fungi, we have the ability to treat patients for a fairly large number of them. Other treatments besides allergy desensitization include topical as well as systemic steroid treatment and antihistamines.

MOLD AND GERD

When you have fungal sinusitis, the toxins can cause enormous mucus production. As this mucus drips into the throat and into the stomach, the stomach will react by producing acid. Typically patients will complain that their noses get clogged up when they are around mold. This sparks their postnasal drip, throat clearing, and coughing. Next, their stomach acids start refluxing. It is thought that this reaction occurs from toxins produced by the eosinophils as a response to the fungal infection which are dumped into the stomach. This may be a similar reaction to feeling like you have to vomit after exposure to food poisoning. The GERD in this case appears to be our body's response to the toxins.

THERE'S MOLD IN MY HOME

Unfortunately, mold is everywhere. Thousands of single-cell fungi are found all over the world. Fungal spores (the reproductive part of the organism) become airborne like pollen. Mold tends to be more prevalent in warm, moist climates but can also be found in cold, dry environments.

Environmental molds are of great concern, as these molds can also cause inflammatory reactions. Dangerous household molds can grow anywhere there is humidity: in the bathroom, in the laundry room, the garage, or the pool area. Mold can be found in the kitchen, in damp carpeting, and in air-conditioning ducts. It grows in basements, barns, movie theaters, restaurants, health clubs, shopping centers, and the garden. For example, Jagger's Manhattan apartment became toxically infested with *Stachybotrys* mold, and she is now fighting for legislation that will help homeowners recoup the expenses of mold removal. *Stachybotrys* causes systemic problems of fatigue, muscle and joint pain, headaches, and weakness. It does this because it incites an inflammatory response in your body.

Often, the warning signs of mold in your home are easy to spot. You can see mold growing on the tiles of your shower, by the sink, or in the washing machine. Other times you may not be able to see it, but can smell mildew. Worse, mold can grow in places that are harder to find, including in plasterboard or drywall and air-conditioning ducts. In these cases, you will need to call in an environmental company that specializes in mold detection.

If mold is found, it is important to have it completely removed. Although it can be expensive, the earlier you address the problem, the less expensive it will be to fix. Typically if you don't fix it, the mold will fester and get worse and it will be harder to eradicate. Unfortunately, there are homes that become so overridden with mold that the house needs to be burned down.

Improving the overall air quality in your home can help you to control your environment and prevent mold growth:

- Use a ventilation system to bring in as much fresh filtered air as you can and consistently remove indoor air pollutants.
- Seal air leaks to block the entry of microbes, allergens, toxins, and irritants.
- Air in your environment should continue to be circulated through filters whether the temperature is warm or cool outside. These filters found in air purifiers; air-conditioners; and heating, ventilation,

and air-conditioner (HVAC) systems need to be cleaned and changed at least four times a year. I change the filters in my home at the beginning of each season.

- Insulate the walls and attic well.
- Vacuum frequently, at least once a week, to remove mold that can be growing in carpeting.

Furthermore, keep your home dry by doing the following:

- Take off wet shoes before walking on carpeting.
- Don't leave wet towels and clothing on furniture or carpeting.
- Purchase a dehumidifier. When the air is very humid, especially in the summer, mold can grow inside your home. This can adversely affect anyone with fungal sinusitis. A dehumidifier placed in strategic locations within the house will help decrease the humidity and the likelihood of fungus growth. Humidity can also cause nasal swelling, and a dehumidifier will help create a more tolerable atmosphere during the humid months of the year.
- The bathroom is the most likely breeding ground for mold. Clean the tiles in and around the shower, sinks and toilets with bleach as it will kill the mold. All wet areas should be dried. Wet towels need to be placed in the washing machine and dried immediately after washing. If you are particularly sensitive to mold, it would be best if you could have someone do this task for you. If not, make sure to have a window open to ventilate the area, and wear a mask.
- The kitchen is another likely location to check for mold. Again, the wet areas need to be cleaned with bleach and should be kept dry. The refrigerator should be cleaned regularly and fresheners should be kept in the refrigerator to keep it clean. Throw out moldy food as soon as possible and wash all of your fruits and vegetables before you eat them.
- Keep all the areas around the washer, dryer and utility sink dry. After using the washer, keep the door open to prevent mold growth inside the washer. Older machines and front loaders are

probably more susceptible to mold growth than top-loading machines. You should run a cycle every couple of days with hot water and bleach to rid the washer of any mold that may start to grow. Remove your clothes from the washer as soon as possible after the wash is finished and place them in the dryer. Keeping wet clothes in the washer is a great place for mold to grow.

- Prevent leaks in your roof and basement. Check basements and attics, and other less frequently used rooms of the house for mold growth on the walls and floors. Mold can also be found growing on upholstered furniture if it is not used regularly.
- Ventilate all areas well to deter mold growth. If outdoor allergens do not trouble you, keep at least one small window open in your home at all times to circulate clean air.
- Keep your car as dry as possible. Vacuum the carpets frequently. In the summer when it is hot and humid, try not to leave wet towels, bathing suits or clothing on the car floor. In any season, when it rains or snows, try to air out your car as often as possible so that mold does not start to grow in the carpet. Make sure that the air-conditioner ducts are dry and clean. Recirculate the air when driving in traffic and when driving on high pollen count days.
- In your garden, do not rake or play in fallen leaves. Cut back the plants that line the sides of your home. There should be a space between these plants and the house so that moisture on these plants does not disturb the shingles on your home. This will also protect your home from water damage.

Avoidance May Be the Key

The good news is that we can prevent mold from affecting your health. Avoidance is often the most important part of treatment. For example, my patient Louise, 61 years old, came in complaining of nasal congestion, bad sinus headaches, a persistent cough, and feeling run down. When I was taking her medical history, she mentioned that there was a leak in her apartment where mold grew around the walls and the floor. She noticed that she felt worse whenever she was in her home, but her landlord refused to clean up the mold, and she could not afford to have her apartment rehabilitated. My first suggestion was that Louise should consider finding a new apartment, but she was reluctant to believe that the mold was the cause of her problems. I started treating her with various medicines and nasal irrigations, and every time she came in I urged her to move. While the treatments helped her symptoms, it wasn't until she finally moved out of her apartment that she improved dramatically.

Treatments

Whatever the cause, be it pervasive mold in your body or in your home, treatment may be necessary. Just as you can get rid of the mold in your home, you will need to rid your body of the fungus causing your immune response. The fungi breeds in the mucous lying on top of the mucous membrane, which can be removed through nasal irrigation with saline or nasal rinsing solutions. By applying an antifungal agent, such as amphotericin B or Itraconazole, to the mucus either through irrigation or a spray, you can reduce the amount of fungi present.

My mold-affected patients spray each nostril twice a day with this antifungal solution. This regimen is known to reduce mucous membrane thickening as well as the related symptoms, thereby reducing the need for systemic steroids. There are few side effects, and this treatment can be used indefinitely, although I usually recommend starting off with a 3-month trial.

A minor side effect of antifungal irrigation, such as Amphotericin B, is a burning feeling in the nose, but this is due to the fact that Amphotericin B needs to be mixed in sterile water. This solution is not easy to obtain: It has to be made at a special compounding pharmacy and must be refrigerated and protected from light. Other antifungal sprays are becoming available to the general public, although this medicine requires a prescription. Because a topical application must get into the sinuses to be effective, it is often necessary to undergo functional endoscopic sinus surgery before it will work with a maximal effect.

Other patients seem to respond to treatment with oral antifungals, including Sporanox and Diflucan. Systemic antifungal agents, such as those given intravenously, have many potentially severe side effects. However, this treatment may be necessary for those with systemically invasive fungus and who are immunocompromised with AIDS or diabetes.

TREATING CAID CAUSED BY MOLD

If you believe that mold is causing your CAID symptoms to flare, you will need to follow the protocols outlined in the other chapters of the book for each specific limb. This may include medical and sometimes surgical therapy. For example, antibiotics are effective in the control of the bacterial infection causing chronic sinusitis. However, antibiotics will not affect the fungi. Over-the-counter (OTC) remedies may offer some relief of symptoms, but they have little effect on the inflammation caused by this reaction to fungus. Certainly, they do not control the effect of the toxins released by the eosinophils. However, the inflammatory reaction can be controlled by nasal steroid sprays, as well as nasal irrigation. Endoscopic removal (débridement) of the fungal material and its secreted toxins has been shown to be beneficial as well.

MAKE YOURSELF LESS ATTRACTIVE TO MOLD

To prevent your body's immune system reaction, you can make yourself less appealing to mold, so it will become more difficult for it to thrive. One important step can be through changing your diet. The foods discussed next are mold magnets: If you can cut down on these items, molds might need to find another more gracious host.

Avoid Sugars and Processed Grains

Fungus feeds on the white stuff: processed sugars and grains (which are simple carbohydrates that break down into sugars through digestion), so reducing or eliminating these foods is necessary to keep fungus under control. I believe that one reason people feel so good on low carbohydrate diets (other than losing weight) is that they are also eliminating the mold growing in their bodies.

Supplement Daily with Cod Liver and other Fish Oils
The omega-3 fats, docosahexaenoic acid (DHA), and elcosapentaenoic acid (EPA) will help strengthen your immune system. Oil-rich fish, like salmon, and dietary supplements including fish and cod liver oils are the richest and most readily available sources of omega-3.

Avoid Mycotoxic Foods
There is a clear relationship between what we eat and how we feel. To my mind, it is quite evident that there is a relationship between foods and the flare-up of CAID. Just as well, there are many foods that are contaminated with mycotoxins (fungal toxins), either in their natural production or from the way they are harvested and stored. These foods are known to increase fungus production within our bodies. It is interesting that all are related to carbohydrates and sugars.

The best results will occur if these foods are completely eliminated from your diet. If that is too difficult, you should at least cut down significantly on their consumption. While it's hard to give up the foods you love, you will probably have a longer lasting joy when you realize how much better you feel than the rush you may get from eating a slice of pizza or chocolate cake. The trade-off is difficult, but it is one of the most important steps in the CAID five-step plan. The food groups of concern include the following:

1. *Alcoholic beverages:* We've already discussed that alcohol is a known problem to sinus patients. What's more, the mycotoxin of the *Saccharomyces* yeast—brewer's yeast—is alcohol. Fruits and mold-contaminated grains are often introduced into alcoholic beverages bringing other mycotoxins to the mix. Therefore, you are probably consuming more toxins than just alcohol in your beverage.

2. *Corn:* Corn is contaminated with fungal mycotoxins. And it's not just the vegetable that you need to avoid: You also need to read labels and stay away from ingredients like corn syrup and corn starch.

3. *All grains:* If it sat in a silo, it stands the chance of being contaminated with fungi and mycotoxins. What's more, grains are used for breads, cereals and pasta. Pasta may be the least "offensive" form of grain, since certain water-soluble mycotoxins float off in the boiling water. Unfortunately, traces of the more harmful mycotoxins remain in the grain.

4. *Sugar (sugarcane and sugar beets):* As discussed earlier, sugars fuel the growth of fungi.

5. *Peanuts:* Peanuts can host up to 24 different types of fungi. Enough said.

6. *Cottonseed:* Packed with mycotoxins, cottonseed is usually found in the oil form (cottonseed oil).

7. *Hard cheeses:* Don't worry about the mold that creates the cheese (blue cheese, Gorgonzola, Brie); instead, worry about the mold that grows on the cheese. Some cheeses, such as Gouda, are made with yogurt-type cultures, which are not fungi.

8. *Fungi as food:* Mushrooms, yogurts, and other mycoproteins should be avoided.

CHAPTER 12

THE LAST RESORT: SURGERY FOR EXTREME CASES

There are times when medications and holistic remedies are not effective enough to make you feel better. For some people, repeated sinus infections or structural abnormalities have created situations in which inflammation and obstruction still exist, even after long courses of medication. In the past, sinus surgery was painful and did not offer great results. However, over the last 2 decades, there has been a great refinement in the medical management and surgical treatment strategies for chronic sinusitis. With newer technology, surgery is much more effective, and safer than ever.

Effective sinus surgery will help you breathe better. In all cases, it will allow the air that reaches the lungs to be filtered, heated, and vaporized, which should improve your asthma and decrease the risk of getting bronchitis and other lung infections. Sinus surgery often provides the sinuses more room to deal with swelling caused by allergies, pollution, infections, and other irritants. If you have allergies, the surgery will not stop the related symptoms from occurring, nor will it change your resistance to infections or sensitivity to pollution and various odors.

However, it can provide significant symptomatic improvement. For example, you may get better results from your allergy regimen after surgery. If you are around children who get sick often, or if your resistance to colds and infections is low, you may still catch a cold or get another sinus infection. However, the surgery will make a cold much more tolerable, and you may not even know that you have an infection.

The surgery should enlarge the natural openings to the various sinus cavities while trying to preserve normal mucosa, leaving as many cilia in place as possible. The goal of the surgery is to return the sinuses to a near-normal functioning state, resulting in the return of normal mucus flow. This essentially allows the sinuses to once again drain properly. If you suffer from sinus headaches, the facial pain due to pressure differentials should improve or disappear. Symptoms of postnasal drip like coughing and hoarseness, stomach upset, sore throat, bad breath, clogged ears, swollen glands, foul tastes, and/or loss of smell and/or taste (unless the olfactory nerve was irreversibly damaged by the infection) should also immediately improve. Surgery will allow you to sleep better because you will be able to breathe better so that you feel rested and alert.

Sinus surgery is also used to remove nasal polyps. In the past, you may have been told that nasal polyps could be removed but that you would require additional surgery about every year or so, and sometimes even more frequently. However, with my comprehensive care program, my patients rarely have to repeat surgery in the operating room. If they can recognize the early symptoms consistent with returning polyps, I can remove new polyps as they begin to return in the office with only topical anesthesia. This technique prevents the polyps from growing too large where they may fully obstruct the sinuses again.

If you had sinus surgery in the past, the newest techniques can offer you new hope for complete relief of your symptoms. It would be a good idea for you to choose a board-certified otolaryngologist—head and neck (ear, nose, and throat (ENT)) surgeon who specializes in revision surgery. A fellowship-trained functional endoscopic sinus surgeon will have the highest level of training, making those few specialists the superspecialists.

When to Consider Surgery

Chronic airway-digestive inflammatory disease (CAID) rarely, if ever, leads to death. Therefore, considering sinus surgery is more a quality-of-life issue than a life-or-death decision. Obviously, for those patients who suffer severely from sinus problems, this surgery can improve their quality of life immensely. Sinus surgery should never be performed for chronic sinus disease without taking the conservative medical approach first. However, there are exceptions, when surgery should be performed as quickly as possible after the initial diagnosis. These instances include the presence of:

- A mucocele
- A papilloma or malignant tumor
- A significant anatomic closure or anomaly obstructing the sinus passageways
- An infection spreading to the eye or brain

COMPLICATIONS TO CONSIDER

Sinus surgery is performed between the eyes and below the brain, so there is a possibility of complication at these sites. Complications of the eyes include visual disturbances, double vision, and blindness. Complications in the central nervous system may include a leak of the cerebrospinal fluid, the fluid that buffers the brain and spinal cord. The incidence of these complications is very rare. Just the same, an untreated infection in the sinuses could potentially spread to the eye or the brain, leading to meningitis or an abscess. The potential of these complications occurring is probably higher if you need surgery and do not undergo surgery. However, when these complications do occur, they can be fatal. In fact, the treatment for a brain or eye infection that is not clearing with medicines in the face of sinus disease is emergency sinus surgery, which does not guarantee any of the untoward effects of these complications.

There is a risk of excessive bleeding, which is just the same as with any type of surgical procedure. However, the latest techniques are far less invasive, and bleeding is usually kept to a minimum. If you undergo a septal procedure, there is a risk of a septal perforation (a hole from one side to the other). Most of these heal by themselves, or if not, can usually be corrected with a small graft at a later date. The septum also has a memory and may return to its precorrected position. More important, as with any type of surgery, there is also a risk of failure. If you are diligent about your postoperative care, the risk of failure, scarring, or recurrence is far lower.

FESS: Functional Endoscopic Sinus Surgery

FESS is an entirely new way to return the nose and sinuses back to their original, anatomical state. I am fortunate to be one of the early practitioners in this type of surgery. It was a privilege to be the first fellowship-trained nasal and functional endoscopic sinus surgeon in the country. I received this fellowship at Johns Hopkins Medical Center while studying under my mentor, the pioneering surgeon, Dr. David W. Kennedy. At the time, many physicians were resistant to the FESS approach. They claimed that Kennedy did not know what he was doing and that his groundbreaking work was nothing more than a fad that would disappear without a trace. Many of my peers ridiculed me for taking the fellowship, claiming that traditional sinus surgery was the way to go.

However, I was more confident. I thought the technology was outstanding. Physicians have used endoscopes as far back as the early 1900s. Kennedy had first learned about these surgery techniques in Europe, and introduced them in the United States. My time at Johns Hopkins Medical Center proved to me that FESS was on the right track; and although I was previously trained as a traditional sinus surgeon, I was completely converted to the other side. I believed that FESS was the way of the future and never looked back.

In 1989, after my fellowship was completed, I returned to New

York. Again, my colleagues snickered. Most of the otolaryngologists were still convinced that FESS was soon to become obsolete. I spoke with my colleagues in general surgery, neurosurgery, and cardiothoracic surgery and advised them to take a look at the endoscopes and apply them in their own fields. They also laughed.

It is now more than 16 years later, and FESS is still considered state of the art. Traditional sinus surgery is rarely practiced, although there are certain indications when it is necessary, and it is still an important tool for sinus surgeons to understand. Today, most new surgeons are trained solely on the endoscope and are taught to perform FESS. What's more, endoscopic surgery is now being performed in almost every other branch of surgery.

I have taught many FESS courses in the United States and abroad. I have had the privilege to teach thousands of surgeons my technique. I am honored that my colleagues have now accepted and embraced FESS, and I am proud to be one of the pioneers.

IS FESS RIGHT FOR ME?

The FESS approach is beneficial to both the doctor and the patient. First, it permits physicians to make a more accurate diagnosis and target the medical and surgical treatment more precisely. After surgery, the endoscopic technique provides the tools to continue treatment right in the doctor's office. During these subsequent checkups, the surgeon can remove persistent, recalcitrant and recurrent infections, scar tissue, and recurring polyps under a local anesthesia. Your surgeon can also directly observe and monitor medical treatment success.

FESS procedures are relatively pain free: most patients need no more than a few Tylenols after surgery. When FESS is performed in the operating room, the surgery is often completed under local anesthesia (therefore obviating the need for general anesthesia and the related risks). An anesthesiologist is always present to administer sedation as necessary. In most cases, the surgery is performed on an outpatient basis, though an overnight stay is occasionally required, especially if you live far from a hospital or suffer from asthma. It is interesting that FESS is usually performed through the nostrils. The surgery rarely requires any cuts on the face, the way that traditional surgery was performed; therefore, there are rarely external scars. The procedure is performed after the patient is sedated with intravenous medicines and then involves an initial numbing of the nose. Then tiny telescopes are inserted along with a variety of microinstruments to remove diseased tissue and obstruction. This allows for appropriate drainage of the sinuses. During the surgery, you may hear a sound like the crunching of eggshells: This is normal and nothing to worry about. Packing is rarely required, and afterward there is minimal bleeding and rarely are there any black-and-blue marks on the face. Patients usually walk out of the hospital and are back to work the next working day. As a matter of fact, I have had patients leave the operating room and go straight back to work, or go shopping.

SURGERY DOES NOT STAND ALONE

FESS is a philosophy whereby your physician or group of physicians and practitioners come together to make a more accurate diagnosis. This occurs by taking an accurate history, performing a thorough physical examination, and then using an endoscope to perform an endoscopic exam to make an accurate diagnosis. Afterward, your physician will develop a treatment plan. Next comes the institution of the treatment, including surgery, if warranted.

Even with the advanced practices of FESS, surgery is only one part of the treatment. In most instances, medical therapy, future endoscopic examinations and treatments, and/or lifestyle changes will still be indicated, even after surgery, to get the best results possible.

You can think of FESS in much the same way we think about treating heart disease. If an obese person requires liposuction to bring his or her weight down and reduce the risk for heart disease, a surgeon will perform the operation. After the procedure, the patient may have lost a total of 150 pounds. However, he or she still needs to exercise and diet, otherwise the patient will end up gaining back all of the weight. Your situation is not that different. If you are a candidate for sinus surgery, even if it is successful, you will still need to take care of yourself, and your sinuses, after surgery.

ANESTHESIA FOR FESS

FESS surgeries can be performed either under local anesthesia with sedation or under general anesthesia. Both have advantages and disadvantages. I prefer to perform FESS under local anesthesia with sedation because I believe that the risks of general anesthesia outweigh the benefits. My patients who have had surgery under local anesthesia with sedation relay that their surgery was well tolerated. Furthermore, patients operated under local anesthesia with sedation can be more easily monitored for warning signs of impending problems. This avoids many of the complications of surgery.

Typically with local anesthesia, there is less blood loss, because the general anesthesia agents cause the blood vessels to dilate. This is a big plus when doing FESS because small specks of blood can look like a red blizzard to the surgeon who is operating through an endoscope. Moderate bleeding can obstruct the surgeon's view and make it impossible to operate safely, necessitating that the surgeon abort the surgery if he or she cannot visualize the operative field.

There are a handful of drawbacks to consider. First, performing surgery under local anesthesia requires more skill than performing surgery under general anesthesia. If your surgeon does not feel comfortable performing surgery under local anesthesia, and you feel comfortable with his or her expertise, follow his or her recommendations for general anesthesia. Your anesthesiologist should also feel comfortable with the technique of providing sedation during this type of surgery. Many are not comfortable and that would be another indication for general anesthesia. However, I've found that most anesthesiologists are comfortable with these techniques.

Nervous or anxious patients might feel more emotionally secure under general anesthesia, although I have found that with proper consultation most are able to easily tolerate local anesthesia with sedation. Children generally require general anesthesia, although I have successfully operated on adolescents whose parents have requested that the surgery be performed under local anesthesia with sedation. If a patient is having a problem tolerating local anesthesia, I can always convert them to general anesthesia during the surgery.

FESS PROCEDURES

Ethmoidectomy

The ethmoid sinuses are shaped like a beehive and are composed of up to 22 smaller cavities or cells. When the anterior ethmoid sinuses are obstructed, typically the frontal and maxillary sinuses will not drain properly, because these two sinuses drain into the anterior ethmoid. This area is known as the ostiomeatal complex. The posterior ethmoid sinuses, if obstructed, can cause significant obstruction to drainage as well.

I specialize in treating patients whose previous sinus surgery has failed. I have found that one of the main causes of a surgical failure is that when the previous surgeon did not open all of the diseased cells in the posterior ethmoid. Retention of residual diseased cells on the lateral wall or the skull base, or failure to properly open the frontal, sphenoid, or maxillary sinuses when necessary can also lead to failure. Scarring in these areas can contribute to a failure, as well as recurrent polyps. It is important that the surgeon be meticulous about ventilating all of the necessary areas which contribute to the disease. Otherwise the surgery is doomed to fail.

There are many schools of thought today regarding which and how many of the ethmoid cells need to be opened. I believe in a conservative approach, preserving as much of the normal mucous membrane as possible while opening all of the obstructed pathways. There are others that call themselves "minimalists"; they believe that you have to open up only a few cells and the rest will take care of itself. Other surgeons will remove all of the mucosa of the ethmoid sinuses, performing a more traditional form of sinus surgery. And then there is the school that still performs a traditional surgery with endoscopic assistance. These surgeons usually remove normal tissue, such as the turbinates, to get better visualization. I come from the school where we are very conservative with turbinate resection and try to preserve the normal tissue whenever possible.

Frontal Sinusotomy

This surgery opens up the frontal sinus, located in your forehead. This procedure is done through the nose in most instances. The passageway up to the frontal sinus is a difficult and technically challenging sinus to open up for most surgeons. I have been sent many cases over the years by other otolaryngologists who are not comfortable with performing frontal sinus surgery. I applaud these surgeons for their honesty with their patients. Less open surgeons might tell their patients that their headaches will go away after an ethmoidectomy, when in fact they have significant frontal sinus disease.

If you suffer from frontal sinus headaches, make sure that your surgeon is confident about operating in the frontal sinus if needed. Often, a clear computed tomography (CT) scan can fool even the best surgeon into thinking that there is nothing wrong in the frontal sinus, but when he or she begins the procedure, the surgeon may find that the passageway needs to be opened.

At times, a surgeon may need to get better visualization of the frontal sinus. A small incision (4 mm) is made by the eyebrow and the surgeon can place an endoscope directly into the frontal sinus. As well, he or she can place instruments into the frontal sinus from above or below and work within the sinus. This incision usually heals without much of a scar.

Failure to open the frontal sinus passageway if required will usually result in the continuation of frontal sinus headaches. The frontal sinuses can be an area where residual infection and disease lingers and then spreads to the other sinuses, leading to failure of medical and/or surgical therapy. Last, if the frontal sinus is not treated properly, a cyst can occur, called a frontal sinus mucocele. This cyst can form 20–25 years after the surgery. Although benign and slow growing, the mucocele eventually erodes the back wall of the sinus into the brain or the bottom wall of the sinus into the orbit (containing the eyeball), pushing the eye off center. I coauthored the first paper on the treatment of frontal sinus mucoceles with functional endoscopic sinus surgery back in 1989.

At that time, most were skeptical. Today, most mucoceles of the frontal sinus are treated with FESS.

Maxillary Middle Meatal Antrostomy Surgery

In maxillary middle meatal antrostomy surgery, the natural ostium of the maxillary sinus is opened. This technique usually obviates the need for the surgeon to remove polyps in the maxillary sinus: it has been shown that they can resolve themselves if normal drainage patterns are returned. However, it is up to the discretion of the surgeon whether to remove any polyps. In any event, if there is an antrochoanal polyp (a polyp that starts to grow from the wall of the sinus and then passes through the opening to the maxillary sinus into the nose), the surgeon should remove not only the polyp as it protrudes into the airway but also the base in the maxillary sinus. Removing this polyp and its base offers the greatest chance of cure. Furthermore, if there is a cyst in the maxillary sinus, the surgeon may want to unroof the cyst, or remove it completely. No matter what the surgeon does during the procedure, polyps and cysts can return or get larger.

Sphenoidotomy

Opening up the sphenoid sinus is one of the most challenging procedures for your physician and requires considerable skill. The object of sphenoid sinus surgery is to open up the natural ostium of the sphenoid sinus. In the case where there is mucosal thickening and/or closure of the natural ostium, opening the natural ostium will provide the necessary relief. However, if you suffer from considerable mucosal disease or formation of a cyst, obstructive polyp or other pathology, the surgeon should address the disease and remove it.

The sphenoid sinus, in competent hands, can be safely operated on. However, many surgeons are uncomfortable with this procedure because the sphenoid sinus is surrounded by many critical structures. The sphenoid sinus sits under the brain and is next to the carotid artery, which carries the blood supply to the brain. An infection in the sphenoid can spread to this artery, and directly to the brain. For this reason, an infection in the sphenoid sinus is very important to treat.

Traditional Sinus Surgery

Most surgeons do not perform traditional sinus surgery any more. However, there are still indications for the traditional approach. The major indications for traditional sinus surgery include the following:

- A mucocele (cyst in the sinus) that cannot be treated endoscopically (most mucoceles can be treated with FESS, although some require external surgery)
- Severe scarring that cannot be removed with FESS
- Infection that cannot be reached with endoscopic techniques
- Inverted papilloma (warts of the sinuses) that cannot be treated with endoscopic sinus surgery (limited papilloma can be treated with FESS)
- Nasal sinus cancer
- When a surgeon is not comfortable treating the disease with FESS

TRADITIONAL ETHMOID SURGERY

Traditional ethmoid surgery is performed either through the nose or through an external incision on the inner aspect of the eye. Packing is usually required, and stitches are placed in the skin at the inner aspect of the eye to close the incision site. The incision will leave a scar and considerable black-and-blue marks around the eye.

TRADITIONAL FRONTAL SINUS SURGERY

Frontal sinus surgery is performed either through an incision by the eyebrow and can be combined with the ethmoid surgery. Occasionally, the surgeon will leave a drain in this area for 24–72 hours, or longer. If the frontal sinus disease is bad enough or the scarring from the disease or previous surgery is obstructive of this area, the surgeon may need to drill out the frontal duct or leave a stent in this area. This procedure combined with an external ethmoidectomy is called a Lynch procedure (frontoethmoidectomy).

For severe disease in the frontal sinus, including a particularly aggressive mucocele, an osteoplastic flap with fat obliteration may need to be performed. This entails an incision across the hair line, where the skin and soft tissues of the forehead are then totally dropped down. The surgeon then can open the frontal sinus, and with fat taken from the abdominal wall, can pack the frontal sinus, thereby obliterating it. Stitches are placed in the forehead to close the incision site and a scar usually remains, which is especially noticeable if you are balding.

There is usually significant swelling and black-and-blue marks to the forehead and around the eyes which usually resolve over a few weeks. Unfortunately, this type of surgery usually means significant blood loss, requires a hospital stay, packing, and general anesthesia.

SEPTOPLASTY

The nose houses many septums, but *septoplasty* refers to an operation on the largest septum, which is the middle part of your nose. This surgery is intended to straighten out the septum so that the airflow through the nose is corrected. This surgery is performed by making an incision into the soft tissues of the septum. The incisions are made inside your nose. The surgeon then lifts the membranes off the cartilage and bone, and then straightens out the septum by either removing or straightening out the cartilage and bone.

I try to preserve as much bone and cartilage as possible, leaving my patients with natural support. Other surgeons remove more of the cartilage and bone and perform what is called a submucous resection. I also try to use endoscopes to perform septal surgery, as it allows me to directly see small deflections without lifting the membranes too far from the supporting septum. I call this an endoscopic septoplasty. I perform most septoplasty surgery with a local anesthesia with sedation, although many surgeons perform this surgery under general anesthesia.

Many surgeons put packing in the nose after a septoplasty. I usually do not and instead quilt the septum with dissolvable stitches.

My patients usually have minimal discomfort and rarely require more than a few Tylenols while they recuperate. In addition, bleeding is minimal and my patients often return to work the next working day. Patients usually remark that they notice an improvement in their breathing immediately after surgery.

Over the next few days you may notice some congestion, swelling, crusting, and scabbing; all of which can be removed at the next office visit. Patients usually remark that their breathing steadily improves after that. They may see slight setbacks with bad crusting and scabbing, which may need to be removed, although usually they find significant improvement in their breathing with a septoplasty.

TURBINATE SURGERY

I believe in being very conservative with the turbinates. Many surgeons just snip or trim off a part of the turbinate. Then there are others that may carry this to the limit by which they remove most of the turbinate. I usually move the turbinate out toward the outside wall. This technique moves the turbinates toward the outside of the airway, purposefully causing scar tissue to the blood supply. This causes the turbinates to shrink, thereby improving the nasal breathing.

If the turbinates are very bulky (called hypertrophied), I perform what I call an endoscopic submucous resection of the turbinate. I do this by making a keyhole incision into the front part of the inferior turbinate and then with an instrument under endoscopic view, lift the soft tissue from the bone. I can then remove part of the turbinate bone, along with some of the soft tissue from the inside of the turbinate, while preserving the outside mucus membranes. Furthermore, I typically cauterize the remaining soft tissue of the interior of the inferior turbinate, and together this causes scarring of the vascular supply and the soft tissues, thereby causing the turbinate to shrink. While the turbinates shrink, I am able to preserve the entire mucus membrane.

I believe that preservation of the external membrane of the turbinate is paramount to getting a good result. Many surgeons cauterize, freeze, and burn the outside membranes of the turbinates. These are accepted methods, but I believe these techniques cause considerable damage to the nose. I furthermore believe that over time less of this type of surgery will be performed and surgeons will be more conservative with the turbinates. However, today many surgeons would argue that removing some of the membranes is just as important to reduce postnasal drip. I disagree. Time will tell, but the pendulum seems to be swaying toward my philosophy.

I very rarely find reason to remove the middle turbinate, except when there is an air cell in the middle turbinate (concha bullosa) that is blocking the nasal airway. The only other time that I resect the middle turbinate is when there is considerable destruction by polyps, although even then, I try to be very conservative with my resection, hoping that I can leave enough of the turbinate so that when it heals it can provide the function of a near normal middle turbinate. Many surgeons resect part of the middle turbinate either with or without a concha bullosa. I believe that this is generally a mistake. Again, the overall philosophy is changing, urging surgeons to be as conservative as possible and try to preserve the middle turbinate.

RHINOPLASTY ("THE NOSE JOB")

Rhinoplasty corrects the overall structure of the nose. It can be performed for cosmetic as well as functional reasons. This surgery can be performed under local anesthesia with sedation or it can be performed under general anesthesia.

Techniques vary from surgeon to surgeon. Rhinoplasty can be performed by making cuts inside of the nose and then tunneling underneath and performing the surgery through these incision sites. Or the procedure can be performed through an external approach (known as external rhinoplasty) through an incision at the tip of the nose, by which the surgeon lifts the soft tissue off of the framework of the nose, giving him or her a direct view of the bone and the cartilaginous framework. I perform rhinoplasties both ways as both techniques have their advantages and disadvantages. I usually decide which way to perform the rhinoplasty based on what needs to be done to achieve the desired functional and aesthetic result. Typically, the soft tissues of the upper and lower lateral cartilages are sculpted with scalpels or scissors, and I like to be very conservative in this area.

During the surgery, nasal bones are usually broken, shaped to the right size, and placed in the right position. However, in doing revision rhinoplasty (after a previous rhinoplasty) rebuilding a collapsed nose after trauma or as a result of an autoimmune disease (Wegener's granulomatosis), bone and/or cartilage grafting may be necessary to build up the bridge of the nose. During functional rhinoplasty, septal surgery is usually performed at the same time for patients whose septum is deviated. Very often the septal deviation lends to the nose being crooked.

Functional rhinoplasty is usually performed when someone suffers a trauma to the nose, which causes a deviation of the nose and leaves it crooked. Trauma to the nose often leads to an obstruction of the nasal airway. This trauma can occur at any time, even as early as coming out of the birth canal. The nose will then continue to grow crooked throughout a person's life. Or trauma can occur as a result of a fall in the crib or a fall when you were young, riding your bicycle, playing a sport, or roughhousing with siblings. You might not remember the incident. Maybe you had a slight nosebleed, a little swelling and the rest went unnoticed. The injuries that you had as a child may not be as apparent as those that occur later in life such as an accident (sports injury or car crash), fall, or assault. Patients usually remember injuries that occur later in life more clearly because they are older and the trauma causes a more acute problem.

There are patients that request a pure cosmetic rhinoplasty. It is important for the surgeon who performs the operation to be cognizant of the fact that changing the outside of the nose can cause nasal obstruction when the surgery is done. Cosmetic rhinoplasty styles change with the times. You can see this by skimming through the fashion magazines. Back in the 1960s many women wanted to have a little, tiny nose. Their plastic surgeon would tell them, "I am going to give you a cute, little nose but I want you to know that your nasal breathing might not be so great thereafter." And the women would say: "No problem, I don't care about breathing through my nose. I just want to look good." Now these women are older and they want to breathe through their nose. In addition, as the years went on, the styles of nasal work changed and the aesthetics of the nose have progressed to a more natural-appearing nose. Now these patients are coming back for their nose to be redone for both functional and cosmetic reasons.

I love doing this surgery and have had excellent results. I enjoy the challenge, and most patients are very appreciative when you can return their nose back to near normal, both functionally and aesthetically. However, some surgeons do not like to do revision rhinoplasty for many reasons, including these:

- It is very challenging and often difficult, even in the best of hands, to get a perfect result.
- It often requires more work and skill than a primary rhinoplasty.
- It often involves an unhappy patient who has had a bad experience with another surgeon.
- The surgery may require significant grafting.
- The surgery may need to occur in stages.

NASAL VALVE SURGERY

Nasal valve surgery is for those who have scarring and/or collapse of their nasal valves. This usually occurs after trauma or as a result of infection and/or previous surgery. When the nasal valve is collapsed or scarred, breathing is compromised significantly. These defects tend to be very difficult to repair and most surgeons do not even want to deal with these defects because of the complexity. The nasal valve area is narrow and scarring tends to recur. Furthermore, when collapse of the nasal valve is a result of a cartilaginous defect in the area of the nasal valve, grafting may be required.

Reconstruction of this area requires significant skill. Flaps may need to be advanced or rotated to prevent crimping in this area. Often this surgery can be performed under local anesthesia with sedation, by directly removing the scar tissue in the nostril, then undermining the area and placing grafts, which act similarly to a collar stay in a men's dress shirt. When more cartilage grafting needs to be placed and rebuilding of the lower lateral cartilages needs to occur, an external rhinoplasty incision may be required.

Lifting the soft tissues off the dorsum of the nose will give the surgeon the visualization that is required to reconstruct the lower lateral cartilages when they are dehiscent (split), scarred, or totally gone. Appropriate support and removal of scar with closure of the wound is required to repair the collapsed nasal valve. Dissolvable stitches are used internally to close the incision sites, and nylon stitches are placed externally (these need to be removed in 3–7 days).

After surgery, the tip of the nose is typically swollen, more so if an external incision is necessary. There are minimal black-and-blue marks, but patients usually have some tape placed over the tip of his or her nose for a few days (up to a week) to keep the grafts from moving. Most of the swelling usually disappears after a few days to two weeks.

Patients are usually able to breathe better immediately after surgery. However, on occasion the surgeon may decide to place a stent in the nostrils, and this can cause some minor discomfort and nasal obstruction. Overall, these stents are removed in a few days to 2 weeks.

What Do I Do about a Broken Nose?

An acute nasal fracture, known as a broken nose, should be reset within the first 72 hours and as soon as most of the swelling goes down. This operation can sometimes be done in an office setting but often requires an immediate trip to the operating room. The surgeon can take an instrument and, without making any cuts, fracture the nasal bones back into proper position. If the septum has been moved as a result of the trauma, the surgeon can also attempt to move the septum by breaking it back into the midline position. This very conservative procedure will most often place the nose back to its pretrauma position and sometimes even move it into a better position than that before the trauma.

This procedure is usually performed with a topical anesthesia and sometimes requires local anesthesia with sedation. If this procedure is not attempted immediately after the trauma (within 72 hours in most cases), the nasal and/or the septal bones will start to heal and fuse in a crooked position. The only option left is for a surgeon to perform a rhinoplasty. I believe it is best to allow time for the bones to heal well before attempting to perform a rhinoplasty. If the bones are not healed, you can increase the risk of shattering the bones, which can be disastrous. I typically wait 3 months or more for the healing process to finish before attempting a rhinoplasty on these patients.

Image Guidance Surgery

One of the latest improvements in nasal and sinus surgery is the use of image guidance systems. Different companies make instrumentation that can calibrate a computed tomography (CT) scan to a machine that hooks up to some of the surgical instruments that your surgeon uses while performing surgery. When your surgeon places these surgical instruments into your nose and sinuses during surgery, he or she can see the position of the instrument on the calibrated CT on the monitor.

This technology sounds like the best surgical thing since sliced bread, and it certainly has been beneficial in many cases. However, use of this instrument is not indicated in every surgery. First of all, the technology has limitations. All of the guidance systems do not connect to all of the instruments needed for sinus surgery. Furthermore, if the calibration is off, the instruments can lead the surgeon into a dangerous area. Use of this instrument adds time to the procedure, and the cost is fairly expensive. Last, your surgeon should use this technology only when it is necessary, and it is important for your surgeon to be comfortable performing the surgery without the instrumentation. The guidance system should be used as an adjunct.

Getting Ready for Surgery

Once you and your ear, nose, and throat (ENT) specialist have exhausted all other medical options, you may be scheduled for surgery. Just like anything else, you need to prepare your mind and body before the procedure. About 2 weeks before surgery, begin following the steps outlined in the following sections. By doing so, you will be creating a healthy environment, thereby increasing the likelihood that your surgery will be a complete success.

STEP ONE

Stop taking aspirin. Aspirin makes people bleed more easily, and surgery patients should not take it for 14 days before surgery and 7 days afterward. If you are taking aspirin, or a medicine containing aspirin, on your own, please stop it, even if it is just a "baby" aspirin. However, if you are taking aspirin on a doctor's order, call as soon as possible and ask if you can temporarily stop. Remember to inform your surgeon of the decision before the surgery date. There is a huge list of over-the-counter (OTC) medications that contain aspirin or blood-thinning substances, including anticoagulants (heparin or Coumadin) and nonsteroidal anti-inflammatory drugs. Make sure you give a complete list of your medications to your surgeon so that it can be reviewed for any blood-thinning substances.

STEP TWO

Continue taking all of your other medications. You must take your sinus medicines religiously before deciding on surgery, so as to give yourself the best possible chance of success. This may actually require 3–8 weeks of medicine (or more), depending on the problem.

Even if you know that you will need surgery, it is a good idea to continue to take these medicines before surgery. The medicines will decrease the risk of inflammation and infection, will lessen bleeding during and after surgery, allow you to heal faster, decrease related pain, and will improve your results.

STEP THREE

Avoid alcohol. Even one beer a day is not good for your sinuses. I suggest that you not drink any alcoholic beverage for 1 week before surgery.

STEP FOUR

Stop taking herbal remedies. Many herbal supplements are contraindicated with anesthesia or surgery. You may think that because these products are from plants, and thus "natural," they cannot be dangerous. Or you may be embarrassed to tell your physician that you are taking something for weight loss, to increase your sexual stamina, clear up your back acne, or fight depression. But remember, your doctor has probably heard it all before. More important, nothing is embarrassing when it comes to safety. Many of these same herbal remedies can be lethal when combined with anesthesia or other medications while undergoing surgery, especially if they have blood-thinning properties. The following is a list of the top anticoagulant offenders:

- **Vitamin E** is usually the number-one no-no. Vitamin E has antiplatelet properties and inhibits vital clot formation. Your surgeon may more than likely ask you to cease consuming vitamin E in any form at least 2–3 weeks before any surgery and for 2–3 weeks afterward.
- **Garlic** (*Allium sativum*), **ginger, alfalfa, cayenne, papaya, feverfew, chamomile, dong quai root, willow bark, goldenseal, guarana, horse chestnut,** and **bilberry** also have antiplatelet properties and may inhibit clot formation.

- **Gingko, gingko biloba, and selenium** are powerful anticoagulants. Each of these are considered to be three times stronger than vitamin E.

STEP FIVE

Eat well and then stop. As with any surgical procedure, a well-balanced diet will increase your chances for optimal results. Good dietary habits and daily multivitamins are encouraged before the procedure, as long as they do not contain the nutrients listed above. You should not eat or drink anything after midnight on the night before surgery, except to take any necessary medicine (as per your surgeon) with a small sip of water.

STEP SIX

Check your overall health. Inform your primary-care physician that you are intending to have surgery. If you have any significant medical problems, you will need clearance from your primary physician. You will need some blood work and if you are over the age of 40, you will need to have an electrocardiogram (ECG). If you are over 65 or have another medical problem, you will need to have a chest X-ray. Every surgeon and hospital/surgery facility has specific protocols of required preoperative testing. It is important to speak with your surgeon at least 2 weeks before surgery to make sure that you are able to schedule all of the necessary tests. Make sure that your surgeon and anesthesiologist get a copy of your testing results before the date of surgery. Furthermore, it is important for you to bring your CT scans to the operating room with you on the day of surgery.

STEP SEVEN

Enlist a friend. Make sure that you have an adult escort to accompany you when leaving the hospital or surgery center. You will not be able to drive immediately after surgery, and many hospitals/surgery centers will not release you without knowing that someone else is taking you home. A taxi is really not a good option. This is the time to call in favors: Remember, that's what friends (and family) are for.

Postsurgical Care

You will most likely be feeling, and breathing, much better immediately after your surgery. However, don't mistake or underestimate the amount of surgery that you have just been through because you feel good. All types of surgery require a healing phase. During this time, it's more important than ever to rest and take care of yourself. When you get home, get into bed. Enlist your friend to stay with you the first night, just in case you don't feel well. Grab a light meal and relax. Take all of the medicines that your surgeon has prescribed for you. Also, take all of your other prescribed medications for asthma, high blood pressure, and so on should you need them. Get a good night's sleep. A vaporizer/humidifier by your bedside, especially during the late fall and winter, may make you feel more comfortable.

The next morning you will probably be slightly congested. You can take a nice warm shower and inhale the water from the shower. The more you inhale, and then either swallow or spit out, the more comfortable you will feel. Put your face in the shower water, turn away and then inhale. Repeat this a few times. You may also wash your hair.

For the next few days after surgery, you may experience some discomfort. The following list of symptoms are all considered to be in the normal range:

- Mild bleeding or oozing
- Mild and possibly moderate sinus headache
- Slight nausea
- Coughing up bloody material
- Nasal congestion

Although extremely rare, immediately notify your surgeon if you experience:

- Visual disturbances
- Severe facial swelling
- Severe unrelenting headaches
- Moderate nausea and/or vomiting
- Eye protrusion or swelling
- Excessive bleeding
- High fever (above 101°F)

BACK IN THE DOCTOR'S OFFICE: FOLLOW-UP CARE

FESS is not over once you leave the operating room. FESS has brought with its development three major advances in the treatment of sinus disease. The first advance is that it has allowed physicians to diagnose sinus disease more accurately. Second, the technique used in the operating room is less invasive and yields greater results. But I believe that the greatest advance that occurred with the development of the endoscope is in the ability to provide immediate postoperative care of the cavity and furthermore provide long-term care of chronic sinus disease. In fact, the postoperative care is almost as important to your overall health as the surgery. I like to think about postoperative care as the care rendered in the first 30–45 days after surgery.

I usually ask my patients to return to my office within the first 3 days after surgery for their first débridement. A débridement is a procedure by which the surgeon removes any crusts, infection, scabs, clots, scar, and residual diseased mucous membranes and/or bone fragments left in the surgical cavity. When my patients come to the office, I first spray their nose with a decongestant and a topical anesthetic. I then use an endoscope and various other instruments to clean out all of the sinuses. It is important to remove as much of the infection, crusting, scabbing and scar/diseased tissue as possible.

The débridement procedure is a little uncomfortable. I usually recommend taking a mild pain reliever or at least a Tylenol about a hour before the procedure is performed. When it is over, you will be able to breathe much better. This procedure is then repeated about once a week for the first month after surgery. The second month usually requires only two débridement treatments, and another one is performed about a month later. For patients with bad chronic disease, long-term periodic débridement treatments with significant medical management may be required.

It takes about 3 months for the sinus membranes to heal to the point at which they are starting to work well and the membranes start to look normal. Débridement may or may not be performed by your physician and some physicians perform more while others perform less. This depends on the severity of your disease, your physician's philosophy, and the type of chronic inflammation that makes you suffer. I believe that patients do best with optimal débridement. The better you control any new infections after sinus surgery by débridement (removal of infected bone and soft tissue and recurrent polyp and scar formation), the better the cavity will heal, the less scarring will occur, and the better you will feel.

On a microscopic level, healing takes much longer. With good care, you should see further progress and greater improvement in your symptoms over the course of the next full year. My patients are usually surprised when they see that the healing phase is not as fast as they thought. Most will continue to see more positive changes occurring over the next 2 years. Overall, it takes about 3 full years to experience the best this surgery has to offer. And it is important that you maintain good health by taking care of your sinuses. Very often, children will not be able to tolerate the débridement cleanings. If your child has had sinus surgery, occasionally your surgeon may recommend that he or she return to the operating room to remove scar tissue/recurrent polyps and debris under either local or general anesthesia.

AT-HOME CARE

Without a doubt, sinus infections can recur. As mentioned earlier, surgery does not change the way you respond to the environment. At best, your sinuses will be near normal. Patients with significant sinus disease can expect that they will continue to get milder sinus infections, usually less frequently. At worst, nasal polyps can continue to grow to where you may still need considerable medical care, chronic care débridement, and possibly revision surgery. When your sinus symptoms flare, you need to address it immediately by seeing your surgeon, so that infection can be removed, along with any recurrent polyps. Your surgeon can decide if you require more medicines than you are taking for maintenance care. No matter where you fall on the spectrum, it is imperative for you to take good care of your sinuses so that they continue to stay healthy.

I often hear my patients complain: "I thought that after my sinus surgery I was never going to need any medicines." As I've already highlighted, this is simply not true. Your surgery does not change the fact that you suffer from chronic sinusitis, and the reason that they call it *chronic* is because it is ongoing and you are stuck with it. In good hands, surgery can make a world of difference, but if you still smoke, are around noxious chemicals, or live or work in a mold-infested environment, then you are going to suffer significantly. Remember, surgery is an adjunct to medicines. To best take care of your sinuses after surgery, you should do the following:

1. Sniff sterile saline water via spray (i.e., Ayr, Goldberger's) and spit out clots as often as possible. The more you wash the nasal cavity with saline, the cleaner it will be. Try to use one entire large bottle for the first 4 days (one 25 ml bottle each day), then ½ bottle each day for the next 4 weeks (approximately 12.5 ml). After the 4th week, I usually have my patients start irrigating their sinuses daily with a neti pot or a nasal irrigation apparatus using sterile normal saline or other preparation.

2. Do not take a bath for at least 1 week. A hot bath may cause your blood vessels to dilate, which can cause you to bleed internally into your nose and sinuses.

3. Take care of your environment. Follow the instructions in the allergy and mold chapters for keeping your house clean and irritant free.

4. Stay away from spicy foods for at least 1 week.

5. Do not do any heavy lifting and refrain from any strenuous activity that may raise your blood pressure for approximately 1 month. This will cause the raw surfaces of your nose to bleed

internally and will generally increase the time it takes to heal. This includes exercising, jogging, lifting, speed walking and long walks, and working out in the gym.

6. No nose blowing for a month. The walls between your eyes, your brain, and your sinuses have been weakened temporarily, and if you create pressure by blowing your nose, you can cause air to be forced into your brain and/or your eye and this can be potentially dangerous. If you feel extremely congested, run hot water in the shower and breathe in the steam and shower water.

7. Sneeze and cough only with an open mouth for 1 month.

8. Gargle with 8 ounces of water mixed with ¼ teaspoon of salt 2–3 times per day for 2 days.

9. Stay away from smoke-filled rooms, fireplaces, and cigarettes.

10. No ocean swimming for 1 month; no pool swimming for 2 months. No diving below the water (either scuba or off a diving board) for about 3 months.

11. You must take all your medicines. One of the biggest reasons for failure of surgery is improper use of medication. I typically have my patients take their antibiotics for 1–3 months after surgery. No matter how long your surgeon keeps you on antibiotics after surgery, you should not skip any doses or stop until you are told to do so by your surgeon. If you run out, you should refill your prescription.

12. You can take Tylenol with codeine or regular Tylenol for pain, if necessary. Stay away from aspirin or aspirin-containing compounds. Approximately 1 week after surgery, restart your nasal steroid spray. If you are taking allergy shots, you should continue with your shots after surgery and not take a break as this may interfere with their success. Any asthma, high blood pressure, or other medicines should be taken as prescribed by your other physicians immediately after surgery.

13. If you were placed on oral steroid tablets around the time of surgery, it is important for you to take them because they will reduce swelling, reduce postoperative pain/discomfort and generally allow you to heal more quickly. These small tablets are

best taken all at once in the morning as they will also usually give you a little extra energy and may make you a little restless at night if you take them in the evening.

14. Sleep on two pillows to elevate your head for at least the next month.

15. If surgery occurs during the winter months, use a humidifier until spring.

16. Continue eating a well-balanced diet and avoid those foods and beverages that upset your sinuses.

Feeling Better, and Loving It

By following the guidelines I've outlined and choosing your surgeon carefully, I believe that you will find significant relief from your sinus problems. Most of my patients report that they feel so much better after surgery. Of course, it is important to try medical alternatives first and opt for surgery only when it is indicated. Many patients put surgery off because they are afraid. Afterward they typically report that their fears were unwarranted. Many have told me that the surgery was much easier than they thought it would be. Typically, they comment that they did not know why they waited so long to have surgery.

For example, my patient Pat was a 41-year-old executive who was debilitated by her sinus disease. She experienced bad facial pain, postnasal drip with yellow-green discharge, and was unable to breathe at night. As a result, she was always fatigued. Pat had already experienced multiple sinus surgeries by other surgeons on her nasal polyps, but they just kept growing back. She said that she never followed any sort of medical care between surgeries. She went to the doctor only one or two times after each surgery and then was discharged and told to come back when there was a problem. When we described our débridement philosophy, she claimed that it was foreign to her. She said that she was suctioned once or twice after each surgery, but that was about it.

I operated on Pat more than 15 years ago, and have kept her on a maintenance course of medicines. Pat follows a healthy diet and exercise

regimen and takes her sinus medications religiously. When she feels a sinus flare-up coming on, she immediately comes back to my office where
I can remove the infection—and any returning polyps—quite easily. Pat
still has occasional headaches, although they are not as frequent and severe, and they are no longer debilitating. She sometimes experiences sinus congestion, but because she takes care of her symptoms with holistic
and traditional treatments, I am able to keep her happy, sleeping well, and
relatively pain free. Pat's experience is much the same as the majority of
my surgery patients, and it can be the same for you as well. You don't
have to live with discomfort or sickness anymore. There is a better life
waiting for you, if you are ready to take the next step.

CHAPTER 13

THE FIVE-STEP PLAN

Now that you understand what is creating your chronic airway-digestive inflammatory disease (CAID) symptoms and have investigated the different treatment alternatives, it's time to put the lessons of this book to the test. The first step is to discuss your findings with your physician, either your primary-care doctor or an ear, nose, and throat (ENT) doctor (otolaryngologist) who specializes in sinus disease. If you find that he or she is not responsive to the treatment plans outlined in this book, it may be that your doctor is not fully informed on the latest treatments and technologies. Science and medicine are ever-changing, and it's perfectly understandable that we all can stand to learn more about our specialties. However, if you find that your doctor is not willing to investigate these treatment modalities, you may want to find another doctor who is more willing to work with you and with these new medical theories. If your physician responds negatively to your newfound knowledge or is obviously uncomfortable working with a patient who is well educated about his or her disease, it's another clear signal that it's time to move on.

Once you've found the right physician, you may need to develop a team of specialists for you to achieve maximum health. This team will be formed to treat your individual symptoms, but may include both traditional and Eastern specialists. Again, look back to your results on the CAID Quiz (p. 70). If you scored particularly high in one area besides the general sinus disease section, make sure that you are including a competent specialist in that field: allergist, pulmonologist, or gastroenterologist. There are ENTs who specialize in these subspecialties, as well as sleep disorders and sleep apnea, and some who fully understand the complexities brought about by mold.

Once your team is in place, your treatment plan should be developed, with everyone on the team onboard. CAID is no less serious than high blood pressure, obesity, and other persistent illnesses: It needs to be managed daily. Your treatment will include all of the various aspects of the five-step plan. By following these five steps every day, you should be able to achieve lasting health.

STEP ONE

Take care of your sinuses through proper irrigation. I cannot stress enough how important irrigation is. Follow the directions given in Chapter 4 every day. Saline nasal spray, the neti pot, and nasal irrigation instruments are very effective. Most of my patients find the procedure for using these instruments to be relatively simple and straightforward, and they seem to love the feeling of clean sinuses thereafter. Daily use of the proper technique yields the best results.

I have had some patients who resisted using nasal irrigation. Some claim that they are afraid to put something in their nose and others are lazy. But without exception, every single patient who has agreed to try using one of these in my office, now uses them on a daily basis. My good friend Gerry, who has been a patient for more than 15 years, finally agreed to try to use the nasal irrigator last year. He came into the office and I went over the technique with him. Since that day, he uses the irrigator daily. He tells me that he loves it and wishes that he started using it years ago. His sinuses are much better as a result.

Whichever method you choose, make sure you give yourself ample time to fully irrigate your sinuses, and then do the stretching exercises so that the irrigation drains completely. Choose a location where you will be able to privately drain your sinuses and then clean up. I find it best to do nasal irrigation in the bathroom during my morning and evening routines. I usually do this at the sink, just before going into the shower (do not use the nasal irrigator in the shower—electric appliances should never be in the shower). I also keep an irrigator at work, and when my sinuses get bad I irrigate in the office bathroom.

In no time you'll quickly learn to master the technique, and once you do, it will come as easily to you as brushing your teeth. Oddly, I often feel that I'm addicted to the procedure, because I feel so much better after I've completed the routine. Immediately, I can breathe easier, my voice is less hoarse, and my throat clearing disappears. As I highlighted earlier, since my surgery, I snore only when I suffer from a bad sinus flare-up. During these bad infections, my wife tells me that my snoring typically disappears if I do my irrigation right before I go to bed. Nasal irrigation is an easy way for you to control your symptoms and alleviate any pain associated with them. It will remove allergens, infections, and pollutants from your airway. Furthermore, it helps wash out infection in the sinuses including viruses, fungus and bacteria. You might find that nasal irrigation is so effective you may be able to stop taking preventative medications, including nasal steroids. For others, nasal irrigation will always be a part of the treatment, and medication or possibly surgery may still be required. And for those of you that have had surgery, nasal irrigation will keep the cavities healthy.

STEP TWO

Clean up your environment. Chapter 5 outlines a plan to free your home of allergens and pollutants. Chapter 11 gives comprehensive information on preventing mold growth and gives tips where to look for mold so that you may be able to remove it from your home, office, and even your car. By combining these two programs, you may find that you instantly begin to breathe easier. You will find that once your environment is more inviting, your symptoms will begin to disappear. That's when you can finally understand the meaning behind the adage, "There's no place like home."

However, a full and stimulating existence cannot be achieved if you lock yourself at home, afraid of dealing with the toxicity found in the rest of the world. When you go out, you may be instantly bombarded with the same allergens, mold, pollutants, and irritants that you have worked so hard to clean up in your homes. I hope that, if you are following the rest of the steps in your treatment plan, you'll find that these irritants should affect you less severely.

For some of us, we may have to reconsider many aspects of your lives to stay healthy. I have had patients that are constantly exposed to irritating chemicals and dusts as part of their jobs. For example, I have patients who are in the construction field, some who work in chemical companies and factories, and others who work in the sanitation field. I have seen teachers, nurses, and even other doctors who are constantly exposed to infection from their jobs. These hardworking people feel as if they had no choice but to live with their symptoms, unless they want to leave their profession. Even I know that my CAID gets better on weekends and holidays when I am not around my patients, but when I go back to work I am around people who are coughing and sneezing near me all day long, and I know that someone will pass along an infection that spurs my sinuses. Yet I love what I do, so I treat myself accordingly to minimize discomfort and continue helping others find permanent solutions for their CAID problems.

There is nothing wrong with the Boy Scout motto: Be prepared. Whether or not you are in a work environment that is making you sick, make sure to carry your emergency medications with you at all times, in case you should have a serious environmental response. If you suffer from allergies, it's a good idea to keep your favorite antihistamines handy, in your purse, pocket, or car. If you suffer from asthma, you should be carrying your beta-antagonist medications like albuterol wherever you go. If you suffer from gastroesophageal reflux disease/laryngopharyngeal reflux disease (GERD/LPRD), you should not leave the house without an antacid that you can take when your GERD acts up. If prescribed, you might want to carry an extra proton inhibitor or an H_2-blocker tablet to take before any large meal. When you return home, remember to wash yourself and your clothes well so that you do not carry these agents back into your otherwise clean environment. By following these precautions, you'll find that you are both emotionally and physically more comfortable visiting new places, meeting new people, and trying new situations. And you'll find, as I have, that these are the small pieces that make life more interesting and enjoyable.

STEP THREE

Be vigilant about food choices. Depending on your particular issues, review the necessary chapters that include information about food and CAID. Chapters 10 and 11 outline nutritional information and foods that should be avoided. Chapter 6 reviews foods that you may be allergic to, or that can affect CAID. Chapter 8 also lists foods that are the most common culprits for GERD/LPRD, while Chapter 9 highlights foods that affect snoring.

It is not surprising that you might have noticed that many of the same foods are the culprits that are causing CAID problems, no matter which symptoms across the limbs of CAID you suffer from. Some of the most common foods causing these problems are carbohydrates (including sugars, grains and alcoholic beverages), dairy, foods containing mold (mushrooms, certain cheeses), and caffeine. In my opinion, this is just one more piece of evidence to support the proposition that these diseases are intimately linked.

It is also interesting to me that these same foods and beverages have been linked throughout history to celebrations, excess, and carefree lifestyles. Could our predecessors have known that these foods cause disease and should only be eaten sparingly? Probably not. Yet in today's culture of easy and inexpensive access to many kinds of food, as well as supersized portions and general overindulgence, we have not learned from experience either. Even though we feel bad while consuming these foods, we continue to eat them. Often, we are our own worst enemies, knowingly eating or drinking something that does not agree with us.

I know that when you first read through the list of no's in any of the food-related chapters, you might have thought that the requirements were overwhelming. I agree: They are. Giving up the foods that you love will be difficult. However, you should see some improvement by simply cutting back on the foods that are causing you to feel bad. For example, I love chocolate cake just as much as the next guy and probably more than even my children. But I know that as soon as I've finished enjoying it, my sinuses will flare. The congestion, postnasal drip and reflux that I experience will quickly surpass the rush I got from enjoying the cake. Ultimately, I know that it isn't worth it.

By far the hardest foods to give up are the grains, because they are found in many prepared foods. I tell my patients to try the elimination diet outlined in Chapter 10 and see how they feel. Afterward, they can reintroduce grains; and if grains are not affecting their health, they may not need to avoid them. However, if you notice a direct correlation after your elimination diet, begin by moderating your food choices so that grains are not in more than one meal a day. If you are still uncomfortable, you may need to take the grains out entirely.

If you require medication for GERD/LPRD, be proactive by taking your medication before meals. If you do, you may be able to widen your range of food choices. Proper nutrient supplementation can also help lessen symptoms and improve your quality of life. If you are considering taking supplements, including naturopathic and/or homeopathic remedies (some of which are listed in Chapter 10), I advise you to seek consultation with a practitioner who prescribes these remedies since their administration for the resolution of CAID is complex. You should also discuss these supplements with your primary-care physician and make sure that your entire team is on the same page.

Supplements often take time to begin working, so be patient. It is important for you to communicate how you feel while taking these products with the prescribing practitioner, as well as with the other members of your health team.

STEP FOUR

Take your medication. I cannot stress this enough: If your traditional or holistic practitioner prescribed medication, take the entire prescription.

Do not stop taking medication just because you feel better or to save pills for another flare-up. Medications, especially antibiotics, continue to work even after the symptoms disappear because the symptoms will often disappear before the infection clears. If you stop taking your medication early, the treatment will be suspended, the infection will not completely clear and—worse—will probably return and may produce resistance.

This is equally important for those who will be prescribed daily medications, including steroid nasal sprays and inhalers. Both of these medications take time to build up their effectiveness: you will probably not see results in less than 1–2 weeks of use. Therefore, don't discard them if you are not getting the results you seek immediately. Instead, discuss your results with your doctor. At this time, he or she might tell you to stay the course or to change medications entirely. The decision will be made based on the information that you give your doctor: Make sure to honestly and clearly explain what you have done in terms of following the directions and how you feel. By working together, you will be able to find the right treatment combinations to combat your particular set of symptoms.

Lastly, remember that even when surgery is the right option, medication might still be necessary for the long term. There is no cure for CAID or any of its chronic limbs. Each are serious and some are potentially life threatening, especially asthma and sleep apnea. Don't fall into thinking that your surgery has cured the disease: Instead it will allow you to deal with CAID as your body starts functioning again on a more normal level. It is really the medication and your body's defense mechanisms that continue to keep your symptoms at bay.

STEP FIVE

Embrace life-altering changes and enjoy your health. If you have begun following the instructions and guidelines in this book, you may already be feeling better. Don't discount your hard work. Change is often both difficult and frustrating. However, if you are miserable, change can literally save your life. You have the power to control how you feel, both physically and emotionally. By continuing your treatment plan and doing the work you need to do to clean up your health and your home, you will reap the rewards, and finally experience what every other healthy person knows: That we should all be able to take our good health for granted.

One Last Lesson: Quit Smoking

Simply being around cigarette smoke or smoking yourself may be part of your problem. Nothing makes my blood boil more than meeting a CAID sufferer who smokes. We all know that smoking is harmful to the body in several ways. What you might not realize is that it is extremely harmful to the respiratory system. Forgetting about your own risks of emphysema and lung cancer, smoking is one of the most harmful things you can do to yourself or a family member that has asthma or sinus disease.

When tobacco smoke is inhaled, the irritants settle in the lining of your nose, sinuses, and lungs and can set off an inflammatory response that can end up as an asthma attack. Smoke also paralyzes, and often literally burns, the ciliated hair cells which are essential for moving these and other irritants out of your body. Study after study has shown that smoking increases the risk of sinusitis. According to one report, people who smoke 11 or more cigarettes a day are about 16 percent more likely to have at least one more case of sinusitis than nonsmokers. People with sinusitis should avoid being around cigarette smoke because secondhand smoke can make symptoms more severe. The report on secondhand smoke speculated that nicotine as well as other chemicals in tobacco smoke may promote sinusitis by affecting the nose and its secretions.

The courts are on my side as well. Entire cities, like New York City, have outlawed cigarette smoking in public spaces, including restaurants and bars. In July 2002, a flight attendant for TWA won a $5.5 million verdict in her lawsuit against tobacco companies, blaming secondhand smoke for her chronic sinusitis problems. The plaintiff was a flight attendant for 14 years before cigarette smoking was banned on airplanes.

SMOKING AND CAID TREATMENT

My position on smoking is clear: You need to quit. However, I know that quitting any addiction is easier said than done. If you currently smoke, clearing up your sinus disease once and for all should be the greatest impetus you'll ever have. First of all, you should refrain from smoking during any treatment for sinus problems. The success of any treatment depends partially on you quitting smoking and may be the number one reason why your previous treatments have failed.

This is especially important when undergoing surgery. If you smoke, to get the best results, you should stop at least 2 weeks before surgery. It is equally important for you to abstain for at least 4–8 weeks after your surgery. Smoking significantly reduces the blood supply to the nasal and sinus membranes. While compromising the blood circulation and impeding vascularity, smoke decreases the amount of oxygen delivered to the tissues, which is necessary for proper healing.

HOW DO I STOP?

There are many effective tools that can be used to quit smoking. But no matter which tools you try, your desire to quit has to come from the heart. If you don't really want to stop smoking, any program will be a half-hearted attempt, at best. So the first step is to get past the defensive denial so that you can face reality. When you finally see how you are truly hurting yourself and those around you, and you decide that it is time to quit, you will finally have a chance at success.

The next step is to find a program that works for you. There are many tools that can be used and many types of physicians and practitioners who work with smoking cessation. I work with a number of them and find them all to be effective. Different therapies will work for different people, and it's often hard to predict what will work best for each of my smoking patients. Your results will greatly depend on your individual personality, level of addiction, and health needs. Don't be afraid to try more than one modality if you do not get good results.

Here are some forms of smoking cessation that you might like to investigate before you start any one program:

- **Medicines.** Usually nicotine substitutes, these include "the patch" or nicotine gums that wean you off of your addition. There are other nonnicotine medicines like Wellbutrin and Chantix that are used for smoking cessation. A traditional doctor must provide a prescription, which will require an office visit and a complete physical examination.
- **Acupuncture.** As described in Chapter 10, this ancient Chinese practice places fine needles on specific meridians or points on the body that will quell the urge to smoke. This requires several visits to an acupuncturist.
- **Hypnosis.** During this treatment you are placed in a hypnotic trance, and your mind is reprogrammed with the subconscious tools necessary to stop smoking. For example, it may be suggested that every time you try to light a cigarette, you suddenly become queasy. The hypnotist, which is often a psychologist, psychiatrist, or holistic practitioner, has created a new response to suppress your addiction. Over time, you will decide that it is not worth the nauseated feeling by choosing not to light a cigarette.
- **Psychological therapy.** A trained therapist can uncover your personal issues that have created a psychological dependency, causing you to smoke. This process also requires many visits to a therapist. Over time, a good therapist not only can get you to see what is causing you to smoke but can give you the tools you need to stop smoking forever.
- **Biofeedback.** This technique uses tiny monitoring devices to gain voluntary control over the desire to smoke. Biofeedback links smoking and other addictions to a stress response. When you are under stress, the monitors can pick up signals your body is sending, so that you can recognize the sensation before you light a cigarette. This program can be done at home, and these products are available without a prescription, either in stores or over the Internet.

NOW WHAT'S HOLDING YOU BACK?

If smoking was your last obstacle, consider that you have taken the first step to get out from under its curse. In fact, just by reading this book, you have taken many, many steps to better health. You now understand how a healthy body should function, and can pinpoint and explain your symptoms. You have uncovered which limb of CAID is causing your discomfort, and you have the tools necessary to create a treatment plan that will work. You are aware of the relationship that mold has with your symptoms. The five-step plan will keep you on track each and every day, so that you can continue to feel well under any circumstances.

My work is done, while yours has just begun. This book provides the information you need to effectively diagnose your CAID symptoms. You now understand that your symptoms may be part of a larger disease process that is intimately connected, including all of the limbs of CAID: sinus disease, allergies, asthma, GERD/LPRD, and snoring/sleep apnea. Best of all, you now have a wide assortment of treatment options and can actively participate in the care of your body.

The sinus revolution has started to bring about a change in thinking on the part of many practitioners that will be taking care of you. You now have the tools to clearly communicate with them. You should feel empowered, knowing that you are part of a team that can resolve your health issues once and for all. My lasting wish for you is simple: That you have found new hope for improvement of your disease, that you really can and *will* feel better.

You can track both your potential diagnosis and treatment options with this CAID flow chart. First, locate your primary symptoms. From there, you will be able to determine which limb of CAID you may be suffering from. If your symptoms are not found in any of the specific disease boxes, check the largest "signs and symptoms" list: If your issues are only found in this box, you are probably suffering from either acute or chronic sinusitis.

Follow the flow chart under your disease path to determine a treatment plan. For many of the limbs of CAID, you might need to see a specialist who will perform further testing to finalize your diagnosis. He or she will guide you to one of the treatment options listed. Start with the least invasive choice, and move to stronger medications or even surgical options if these are not successful. Be open to trying both Eastern and Western remedies, and speak with your treating practitioner to see what is available and appropriate for your specific issues. By following your personalized treatment plan, you can easily become symptom-free.

Many times CAID symptoms will overlap, and you might find that you are simultaneously experiencing more than one limb of CAID. For instance, you might be suffering from both allergies and asthma, or snoring and chronic sinusitis. CAID symptoms can also manifest new disease processes. For example, chronic postnasal drip is a symptom of sinusitis and can cause GERD to flare up. Allergies can also cause chronic sinusitis. Hoarseness and chronic coughing can be caused by either chronic sinusitis or LPRD/GERD, or both.

Once you understand the intricate connection between your symptoms, you will be able to help your physician/practitioner both accurately diagnose and then treat each of your disease processes. By doing so, your health will improve and you will start to feel better.

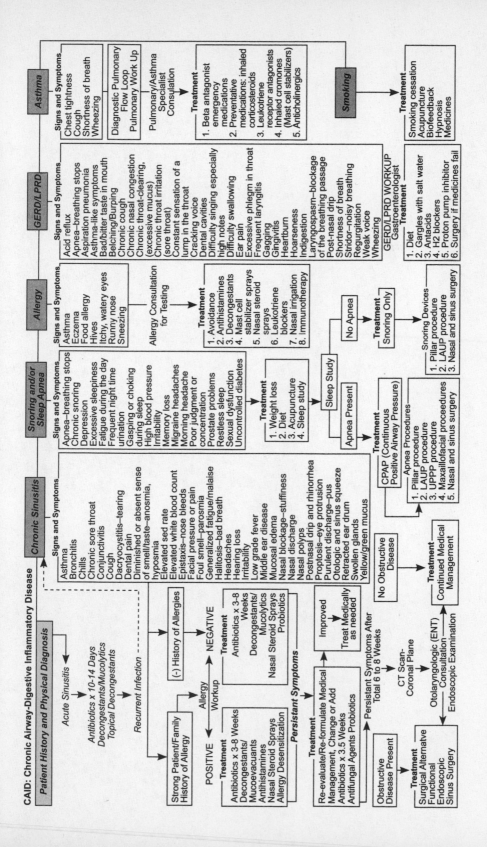

CAID: Chronic Airway-Digestive Inflammatory Disease

Patient History and Physical Diagnosis

Chronic Sinusitis

Acute Sinusitis

Antibiotics x 10-14 Days
Decongestants/Mucolytics
Topical Decongestants

Recurrent Infection

Signs and Symptoms
Asthma
Bronchitis
Chills
Chronic sore throat
Conjunctivitis
Cough
Dacryocystitis–tearing
Dental pain
Diminished or absent sense of smell/taste–anosmia, hyposmia
Elevated sed rate
Elevated white blood count
Epistaxis–nose bleeds
Facial pressure or pain
Foul smell–parosmia
Generalized fatigue/malaise
Halitosis–bad breath
Headaches
Hearing loss
Irritability
Low grade fever
Middle ear disease
Mucosal edema
Nasal blockage–stuffiness
Nasal discharge
Nasal polyps
Postnasal drip and rhinorrhea
Proptosis–eye protrusion
Purulent discharge–pus
Otologic and sinus squeeze
Retracted ear drum
Swollen glands
Yellow/green mucus

(-) History of Allergies

Allergy Workup

NEGATIVE

Treatment
Antibiotics x 3-8 Weeks
Decongestants/
Mucolytics
Nasal Steroid Sprays
Probiotics

Strong Patient/Family History of Allergy

POSITIVE

Treatment
Antibiotics x 3-8 Weeks
Decongestants/
Mucoevacuants
Antihistamines
Nasal Steroid Sprays
Allergy Desensitization

Persistant Symptoms

Treatment
Re-evaluate/Re-formulate Medical Management, Change or Add
Antibiotics x 3.5 Weeks
Antifungal Agents Probiotics

Improved

Treat Medically as needed

Persistant Symptoms After Total 6 to 8 Weeks

CT Scan-Coronal Plane

Otolaryngologic (ENT) Consultation
Endoscopic Examination

Obstructive Disease Present

Treatment
Surgical Alternative
Functional
Endoscopic
Sinus Surgery

No Obstructive Disease

Treatment
Continued Medical Management

Snoring and/or Sleep Apnea

Signs and Symptoms
Apnea–breathing stops
Chronic snoring
Depression
Excessive sleepiness
Fatigue during the day
Frequent night time urination
Gasping or choking during sleep
High blood pressure
Irritability
Memory loss
Migraine headaches
Morning headache
Poor judgment or concentration
Prostate problems
Restless sleep
Sexual dysfunction
Uncontrolled diabetes

Treatment
1. Weight loss
2. Diet
3. Acupuncture
4. Sleep study

Sleep Study

Apnea Present

No Apnea

CPAP (Continuous Positive Airway Pressure)

Treatment Apnea Procedures
1. Pillar procedure
2. LAUP procedure
3. UPPP procedure
4. Maxillofacial proceedures
5. Nasal and sinus surgery

Treatment Snoring Only

Snoring Devices
1. Pillar procedure
2. LAUP procedure
3. Nasal and sinus surgery

Allergy

Signs and Symptoms
Asthma
Eczema
Food allergy
Hives
Itchy, watery eyes
Runny nose
Sneezing

Allergy Consultation for Testing

Treatment
1. Avoidance
2. Antihistamines
3. Decongestants
4. Mast cell stabilizer sprays
5. Nasal steroid sprays
6. Leukotriene blockers
7. Nasal irrigation
8. Immunotherapy

GERD/LPRD

Signs and Symptoms
Acid reflux
Apnea–breathing stops
Aspiration pneumonia
Asthma-like symptoms
Bad/bitter taste in mouth
Belching/Burping
Chronic cough
Chronic nasal congestion
Chronic throat-clearing, (excessive mucus)
Chronic throat irritation (sore throat)
Constant sensation of a lump in the throat
Cracking voice
Dental cavities
Difficulty singing especially high notes
Difficulty swallowing
Ear pain
Excessive phlegm in throat
Frequent laryngitis
Gagging
Gingivitis
Heartburn
Hoarseness
Indigestion
Laryngospasm–blockage of the breathing passage
Post-nasal drip
Shortness of breath
Stridor–noisy breathing
Regurgitation
Weak voice
Wheezing

GERD/LPRD WORKUP
Gastroenterologist

Treatment
1. Diet
2. Gargles with salt water
3. Antacids
4. H2 blockers
5. Proton pump inhibitor
6. Surgery if medicines fail

Asthma

Signs and Symptoms
Chest tightness
Cough
Shortness of breath
Wheezing

Diagnostic Pulmonary
Flow Loop
Pulmonary Work Up

Pulmonary/Asthma Specialist Consultation

Treatment
1. Beta antagonist emergency medications
2. Preventative medications: inhaled corticosteroids
3. Leukotriene receptor agonists
4. Inhaled cromones (Mast cell stabilizers)
5. Anticholinergics

Smoking

Treatment
Smoking cessation
Acupuncture
Biofeedback
Hypnosis
Medicines

INDEX

Dr. Jordan S. Josephson is the director of the New York Nasal and Sinus Center. Selected as one of *New York* magazine's "New York's Best Doctors" in 2004 and 2006 and featured as one of the magazine's "13 Innovators in Medicine," Dr. Josephson is an internationally recognized nasal and endoscopic sinus surgeon. He is also a sinus, asthma, and allergy sufferer who is committed to finding the most effective treatments for adults and children. Embracing both traditional medicine and successful alternative therapies, he has become one of the country's leading experts on sinus disease, allergies, asthma, gastroesophageal reflux disease (GERD), snoring/sleep apnea, and nasal deformities leading to airway obstruction. He is also recognized as an expert in functional endoscopic sinus and nasal surgery.

Dr. Josephson's New York office is affiliated with prestigious institutions, such as Lenox Hill Hospital and Manhattan Eye, Ear & Throat Hospital. Beyond the traditional clinical treatment of his patients, he actively participates in the latest research and uses this knowledge as a medical educator, lecturing around the world. In 2004, Dr. Josephson was given the honors award by the American Academy of Otolaryngology—Head and Neck Surgery, the largest professional organization of his specialty in the world.

Dr. Josephson received his undergraduate degree with distinction from the State University of New York at Albany and attended the State University of New York at Downstate Medical School. He completed his internship in general surgery and then focused on a specialized residency in otolaryngology at Long Island Jewish Hospital, where he finished as chief resident. Dr. Josephson was then chosen to become the first fellowship-trained nasal and functional endoscopic sinus surgeon in the United States. He completed this fellowship at the Johns Hopkins Medical Center, where functional endoscopic sinus surgery was first introduced in the United States. At the Johns Hopkins Medical School, Dr. Josephson held the rank of instructor.

Based on his research, Dr. Josephson was asked to consult for the National Institutes of Health (NIH) on the most cutting-edge work in this field. He worked with the NIH for 7 years doing research and providing clinical care to patients with sinus disease and nasal and facial collapse who suffered from unusual immune disorders. Dr. Josephson pioneered special grafting techniques for reconstruction of the nose and midface in these patients. In 1994, he received the prestigious service and dedication award from the NIH for his efforts in research and patient care.

Dr. Josephson has taught hundreds of doctors and surgeons on the delicate operative techniques of functional endoscopic sinus and nasal surgery. He has been invited to teach as an honorary guest lecturer across the globe, and his articles and chapters on the subject of functional endoscopic sinus surgery and facial cosmetic surgery have been published in many languages. He has authored and edited two books for the Medical Clinics of North America, which are published in five languages and are a staple of most hospital libraries around the world.

Dr. Josephson regularly appears as a medical expert on various national and local television programs. He has been featured on a variety of news programs on CBS, NBC, CNN, FOX, including *The Today Show*. He has been featured and quoted in magazine and newspaper articles, including the *New York Times*, *New York Post*, *Newsday*, *Newark Star-Ledger*, *Medical Herald*, *Boston Globe*, *Alert Diver*, *Bottom Line/Health*, *Allure*, *Men's Health*, *Parenting* magazine, *Bicycling*, and *Elle*. He has been interviewed on websites such as DiscoveryHealth.com, CNN.com, and BottomLineSecrets.com. Visit his website at www.drjjny.com.

THE SINUS AND NASAL INTERNATIONAL FOUNDATION (SNIF)

Dr. Josephson, along with a team of related physicians, has formed the Sinus and Nasal International Foundation (SNIF), a patient organization with a coalition of doctors and worldwide opinion leaders who advocate providing comprehensive education for people with sinus disease, allergies, or asthma. Dr. Josephson currently serves as the chairman of the board of this foundation.

The goal of SNIF is to standardize the health-care approach for those who suffer from these related illnesses. SNIF aims to establish treatment protocols throughout the world, create community and patient educational programs, and encourage research into the causes of these diseases. SNIF's professional team represents every facet of twenty-first century medicine: traditional specialists—ear, nose, and throat specialists; allergists; pulmonologists; internists; primary-care specialists; and family practitioners—working in concert with many of alternative medicine's finest osteopaths, naturopaths, acupuncturists, and chiropractors, among others.

For more information, visit www.snif-us.org.

Sinus Relief Now

Please visit www.sinusreliefnow.com for new material and the latest information on topics covered in this book.